98305
8-

ANNALS OF THE NEW YORK ACADEMY OF SCIENCES

VOLUME 169 ARTICLE 3 PAGES 595–738

June 23, 1970

THIRD CONFERENCE ON THE FUNDAMENTALS OF PSYCHOLOGY: VARIOUS APPROACHES TO THE STUDY OF PERCEPTION*

Editors and Conference Cochairmen

ERNEST HARMS AND MARGARET E. TRESSELT

CONTENTS

Opening Remarks. *By* ERNEST HARMS

Part I. Perception of the Outer World

Visual Information Processing with Sequential Inputs: A General Model for Sequential Blanking, Displacement, and Overprinting Phenomena. *By* M. S. MAYZNER AND M. E. TRESSELT 599

Complexity and Preference in Animals and Men. *By* EDWARD L. WALKER 619

The Perception of Gestalt–1969. *By* HARRY HELSON 654

Part II. Perception of the Inner World

Inner Perception in Terms of Depth Psychology. *By* JOSEPH L. HENDERSON 664

Perceiving and Thinking: Their Interrelationship and Organismic Organization. *By* WALTER S. BOERNSTEIN 673

The Self, Reality, and Perception. *By* LEO A. SPIEGEL 683

Perception–Yesterday, Today, and Tomorrow. *By* ERNEST HARMS 694

Part III. Perception in Abnormal Psychological Experience

Role of Perception in Identifying Psychopathology. *By* MAURICE LORR 697

Changing Relations of Symptom Perception to Psychoanalytic Therapy. *By* BENJAMIN WOLSTEIN 706

Perceptual Functioning in Schizophrenia: Implications for the Study of Perceptual Processes. *By* IRVING B. WEINER 718

Part IV. Perception of Creativity

The Perception of Objects of Art. *By* CARROLL C. PRATT 731

Concluding Remarks. *By* MARGARET E. TRESSELT AND ERNEST HARMS 737

* This series of papers is the result of a conference entitled Various Approaches to the Study of Perception, held by The New York Academy of Sciences on October 13 and 14, 1969.

OPENING REMARKS

Ernest Harms, Ph.D.

This is the fourth conference on the fundamentals of psychology conducted during the past ten years, and the third to take place at the Academy of Sciences. The purpose of these conferences has been to help solidify and clarify basic concepts in the field of psychology, which has grown to such an enormous degree during the past decades that no one, as we all know, could alone keep up with the publications that are constantly appearing. However, it should concern us still more that the entire field seems to have lost its basically sound perspectives and been unable to coordinate the work done by various groups in numerous specialized disciplines. I earlier used the symbolic image of the Tower of Babel to describe the condition of our field of endeavor; this "tower" continues to grow from year to year, and hardly anything is being done to remedy the conditions.

In this conference we wish to review basic concepts, and we shall attempt a thorough discussion about the present status, propose a new solid frame, and inaugurate good coordination for the perception factor. Our previous conferences on thinking, the ego, and emotions and feelings have proven to have made an astonishingly deep and strong impact in the field. That we have chosen the subject of perception for this new conference is, I may say, only natural. Considering the importance of perception in the field of psychology, it should have been the first topic. However, even we must confess that we are subject to various impulses. And I hope that this two-day conference will serve to correct our earlier omission.

Someone once called perception the "creation myth" of the science of psychology. He no doubt wished to emphasize that perception is the first basic element to be considered and should be taken up first in a scientific study of the human psyche. An historical survey will show us that as far back as we are able to go in the observation and study of human personal experience, perception was considered fundamental. When scientific psychology was begun during the early period of the past century, we find that perception study was given first place. Herman von Helmholtz, the master architect of our field, planted, in his superb works on visual and acoustic perception, the pillars for the basic structure. Most of his basic concepts are still valid, and what he once started has not ceased to be the major concern of psychologists. No one has yet attempted a history of the development of the perception concept to the present, showing the variety of interpretations and the confusion in regard to them. A bird's eye view of perception, as it is presented in our present literature, calls for a comparison with a Middle-American virgin forest in which the great originals of a past culture are buried beneath the undergrowth. We are here, however, not for historical study, but to try to clear the ground, pointing out what is essential, and setting up guidelines for future exploration.

A conference like this, composed of a dozen or so lectures, must limit itself to an outline program. We have made the most of this forced limitation. In evaluating a major portion of present perception studies, one will have to realize that the concept of self-perception is by far the most dominate. If we apply a more fundamental view, this must appear rather limited and limiting. Along with the tremendous widening of the application of psychology, as experienced during recent decades, a widening of the conceptional sphere of perception has also taken place. Perception is no longer merely sense-perception. We feel this is an issue of utmost importance, important enough, in fact, to be made the basic theme of this conference. To preview in short: the concept of perception we apply in the thinking process, on emotions and feelings, in the field of the mentally and psychologically abormal, and finally in regard to creative processes in the cultural world, definitely has a character different from that of the sense perceptions as it was formulated by Helmholtz. We are tackling here a task which makes us pioneers and "advance scouts." If we can prove that we are right, we will be forced to challenge the science of psychology and insist on a considerable revision and broadening of the field of perception. We are calling for a considerable amount of new study and research. This will be a great ncw task for psychology. Let us go ahead with it.

PART I. PERCEPTION OF THE OUTER WORLD

VISUAL INFORMATION PROCESSING WITH SEQUENTIAL INPUTS: A GENERAL MODEL FOR SEQUENTIAL BLANKING, DISPLACEMENT, AND OVERPRINTING PHENOMENA*

M. S. Mayzner, Ph.D. and M. E. Tresselt, Ph.D.†

New York University, New York, N. Y.

Introduction

There would probably be little disagreement that one of the most complex and challenging problems in the area of visual perception is a specification of the mechanisms by which the visual system deals with space-time interactions. Such interactions have been studied intensively, over many decades, with a variety of research strategies. Problems of flicker, intermittent stimulation, and apparent movement,[11,36] problems of visual masking[17] the current surge of interest in Mach bands[30] all attest to the methodological diversity that characterizes the study of space-time interactions in the visual system. Certainly a better understanding of such interactions would contribute materially to our overall knowledge of general visual system performance.

What is the most effective approach to the problem of space-time interaction? If we conceptualize the visual system as an information processing system, which has recently become a common strategy in visual research,[7,31] with a given processing capacity, then it becomes reasonable to expect that overloading this processing capacity may produce space-time interactions. For example, the most general paradigm for such overloading is to present the visual system with a pair or a string of sequential stimuli or inputs at a display rate that exceeds, the system's spatio-temporal resolving power. If a pair of stimuli is employed, some form of visual masking is typically implicated, while with a string of stimuli, interest is usually focused on such issues as the display rate that produces fusion, or on those display parameters that produce an experience of apparent movement. In all of these cases of space-time interactions, the central distinguishing feature is a breakdown of the visual system to provide an output that represents a veridical and isomorphic match to the input. In visual masking paradigms, space-time interactions are revealed by failures of the *S*'s visual output to match the input, such that, depending on the parameters under investigation, one or both of the inputs may be misperceived, or one input may not even be detected. With strings of stimuli, other types of input-output mismatches may occur, such that if the display rate is high enough and all the stimuli occur at the same location in space, total fusion will occur, or if the stimuli are displayed at different locations, all the stimuli will appear as if they have been displayed simultaneously, when, in fact, they have been displayed sequentially. In brief, space-time interactions can produce a rich variety of input-output mismatches, for example: (1) failures of stimuli to be detected, (2) failures in the ability to detect sequential orderings of stimuli, (3) distortions in the spatial locations of stimuli, (4) distortion in the sharpness, clarity, or apparent duration of stimuli, (5) distortions in the relative subjective brightness of stimuli, (6) various experiences of apparent movement, and so on.

* This research was supported by grant no. GB–8037 from the National Science Foundation to the senior author.

† The sudden and untimely death of Dr. Tresselt was much to be regretted during production of this monograph. – Ed.

The present paper will be directed primarily towards three perceptual phenomena that exhibit marked space-time interactions and the associated input-output mismatches that occur with such interactions, which we have been studying intensively over the past three years. These are "sequential blanking," "sequential displacement," and "overprinting" phenomena. We shall also be concerned with developing a general model of visual information processing designed to conceptualize these phenomena within a single theoretical framework. We have chosen these three particular phenomena to focus upon since they exhibit marked space-time interactions rarely observed or studied before because of previous display hardware limitations. It seems appropriate, therefore, before proceeding with the substantive portion of our paper, to describe briefly our current hardware configuration, which will perforce indicate previous hardware limitations and also disclose the very great flexibility of our current hardware system for the study of space-time interactions in the visual system.

Hardware System

Our current hardware system consists basically of a computer-based cathode-ray tube (CRT) display system. Very briefly, this system consists of a high-speed PDP-7 digital computer, which, when appropriately programmed, will display alpha-numeric characters, point light sources, or geometric configurations on some four CRT display consoles interfaced to the computer. The display surfaces of three of the CRT consoles are coated with an ultra short persistence phosphor (P24), having a decay time on the order of a few microseconds (μsec). This essentially instantaneous decay of phosphor excitation coupled with a 20 kHz crystal clock within the computer permits input display times to go as low as 50 μsec per input and to vary upwards in 50 μsec increments. Inputs may be spatially located wherever desired on the CRT display surface. Thus, this display system provides an extraordinary degree of space-time flexibility in the display of input configurations, far beyond typical display devices of the past, such as tachistoscopes and various types of optical projection systems. A fuller description of this display system may be found in our previous papers.[20,24]

Associated with this hardware system is a set of highly flexible display programs, which allows the experimenter to construct, by means of teletype or typewriter inputs, an almost infinite variety of display configurations. For example, with our present display programs, any member of an alpha-numeric character set (i.e., any of the characters found on a typical typewriter keyboard, such as letters, digits, and such special characters as —, /, +, =, !, etc.) may be displayed in any one of the 1,600 cells of a 40 × 40 cell matrix. This allows for a wide variety of display configurations, such as horizontal arrays, vertical arrays, oblique arrays, and any combinations thereof, and the number of individual inputs or characters displayed may vary from one to 100. The 100 individual inputs can all be displayed sequentially, i.e., one character at a time, each in a different cell of the 1,600 cell matrix, or if desired, they may also be displayed all in one cell, one input after another, or any mix of same or different cells desired. Further, subsets of characters may be displayed simultaneously, while preserving sequentiality between subsets. Also, any mix of subsets and subset sizes may be displayed in any order, display location, and input rate desired.

In addition, other display programs allow for the display of up to 100 point light sources or up to 100 straight-line segments, in a manner equivalent to the options available with the alpha-numeric program. In brief, this hardware display system and its associated computer programs (software) allow an experimenter to construct almost any type of display configuration desired very quickly and very easily by simply typing in on the computer teletype console the desired display parameters.

Research Terminology and Strategy

As we have already indicated, we shall be concerned in this paper with certain types of space-time interactions that occur in the visual system. In a recent review of such space-time interactions, as found in visual masking paradigms, Kahneman[17] indicates that the term "visual masking" appears to have been first used by Pieron[29] and "covers the class of situations on which some measure of the effectiveness of a visual stimulus (the test stimulus, TS) is reduced by the presentation of another (the masking stimulus, MS) in close temporal contiguity to it." (p. 404) Kahneman further distinguishes between forward and backward masking, i.e., when MS precedes TS or when TS precedes MS, respectively. Typically, in such forward and backward masking paradigms, TS and MS spatially superimpose or overlap each other in space. When TS and MS do not spatially superimpose or overlap each other, but rather, occupy adjacent locations in space but again in close temporal contiguity, the terms forward and backward masking are usually replaced by terms introduced by Stigler[34] some 60 years ago, namely, paracontrast and metacontrast, respectively.

It is critical to note that in the visual masking nomenclature just outlined and in the over 100 studies of visual masking and metacontrast reviewed by Kahneman, almost every study examined employed experimental paradigms involving only two stimuli or inputs to the visual system. In sharp contrast, our research strategy[24] for studying space-time interactions in the visual system involves presenting to the visual system increasingly longer and more complex spatio-temporal input configurations. It would be our position, in fact, that a two-input string to the visual system represents a highly special and highly limiting case of potential space-time interactions in the visual system, and the work to be reported in this paper supports this view.

More specifically, with the display system we have been employing, for the first time it has become possible to present to the visual system highly complex spatio-temporal input configurations, which, in turn, allows for the study of sequential blanking, displacement, and overprinting phenomena. For example, the letters that make up the word "SOMERSAULT" are displayed sequentially in their appropriate spatial or individual letter locations on a CRT display console. With ten letters displayed sequentially, in ten adjacent spatial locations, there are 10!, or 3,628,800 different display orders possible. In TABLE 1, the word "SOMERSAULT" is shown along with a few selected input display

TABLE 1

SELECTED DISPLAY ORDERS FOR "SOMERSAULT"

	Sequence									
Display	S	O	M	E	R	S	A	U	L	T
Orders	1	2	3	4	5	6	7	8	9	10
	10	9	8	7	6	5	4	3	2	1
	1	3	5	7	9	2	4	6	8	10
	7	5	9	2	1	10	4	3	8	6
	1	6	2	7	3	8	4	9	5	10

orders, as given in the lines of numbers under the word, such as 12345678910, 10987654321, 13579246810, 75921104386, and 16273849510, with each number indicating the sequential ordering of the letters being displayed. Thus, with the first two display orders, the letters are displayed sequentially in order from left to right or right to left, respectively, while with an order such as 75921104386, "R" is displayed first, "E" second, "U" third, "A" fourth, and so on. In the last two lines of the display orders shown, certain numbers have been underlined, which means that if appropriate input rates are employed (i.e., 10 msec "on" per letter and 10 msec "off" between letters, or 1 msec "on" and 19 msec "off" or 19 msec "on" and 1 msec "off," or, in fact, any "on-off" time combination yielding a total of 20 msec per letter or a total display time of 200 msec for all 10 letters), *S*'s typically report the underlined letter locations as being totally empty, showing a slight blur of light, or with very intense fixation on a missing letter location, a very dim percept of the letter falling in that position. This effect we have called sequential blanking.[23,25] One might note in passing that with display orders 1–10 or 10–1, no blanking is reported with all ten letters clearly perceived.

With the display order 13579246810, and at input display rates that produce sequential blanking effects, the phenomena we have called sequential displacement occurs.[25,26] In sequential displacement, all *S*s report clearly perceiving all ten letters, but are convinced that a wide empty space about a letter-to-two-letter widths in extent occurs between the letters displayed ninth and second, i.e., between "R" and "S."

In studying overprinting phenomena,[25] rather than displaying inputs sequentially at different spatial locations on the CRT display surface, all inputs are displayed in the same spatial location. For example, with the overprinting paradigm, one might choose to display the letters of "SOMERSAULT," one on top of another, or a string of digits, one on top of another, or a string of words, one on top of another.

Having briefly outlined the three general types of space-time interactions we shall be concerned with, and before discussing their theoretical implications for a visual information processing model, we should like to indicate that our particular choice of terminology was deliberate and not designed to introduce still more new terms into the perceptual literature, without, we believe, a basically sound rationale. It is our position that while para- and metacontrast involve the display of inputs in adjacent spatial locations, as does our sequential blanking and displacement phenomena, historically, para- and metacontrast have been concerned exclusively with a two-input string. A two-input string is, in our view, merely a special and rather limiting case of an N-input string, and therefore, para- and metacontrast are merely subsets of the far more general space-time interactions we have called sequential blanking and sequential displacement. Further, forward and backward masking, in which inputs superimpose or spatially overlap one another, and which fall under the more general rubric of visual masking, again have historically been concerned with only the restrictive subset of two-input strings, with few exceptions,[32] while the term overprinting is needed to refer to the more general N-input string paradigm.

The General Model: Sequential Blanking and Displacement Effects

Since Broadbent's[5] (1958, p. 299) "information-flow diagram for the organism," there have been increasing attempts to conceptualize the "route" or "pathway" through the organism that links input or stimulus to output or response. In this tradition we recently proposed[25] a provisional model of visual information processing with sequential inputs, and FIGURE 1 presents an information-flow diagram of this model. Very briefly, this model suggested that when a string of sequentially displayed visual inputs (whose "on" time varies from 50 μsec to approximately 50 msec and are clearly above threshold) enters the visual system, the inputs pass through a succession of information or data processing components, i.e., visual receptor mechanisms, visual cortex, higher centers (central storage), a gating mechanism, and finally arrive, after about 130 msec of real-time input processing, at a component we have called "subjective visual experience" (SVE). This component represents the *S*'s actual subjective visual experience associated with any given visual input, which is above threshold and whose duration, or "on" time, varies from 50 μsec to about 50 msec. Further, we estimated input processing time in SVE to be on the order of about 100 msec, which has subsequently been confirmed in a more recent study[35] and also agrees very well with similar types of estimates made by other investigators.[8,10,18] We also suggested that visual inputs, once having passed through SVE, may enter a "rehearsal loop" which feeds into the central storage component of the model, and where subsequent retrieval mechanisms operate on the inputs, making them available for verbal report.

In this provisional model, because of our concern with space-time interactions, we explicitly attempted to identify a "real-time processing value" for each of the major data processing components of the model, as indicated along the time base. For example, a string of inputs begin to impinge on the retina at time t = 0; certainly no SVE would occur at this instant or even 10 to 20 msec later, since in this connection Woodworth and Schlosberg[37] state, "When a light is thrown into the eyes, activity reaches the visual cortex in 20–40 msec." (p. 19) Should we even assume that SVE occurs at t = 30 or 40 msec? This seems unlikely, but raises the question of just how much time is required for real-time input message processing before the SVE component is reached. An upper bound is fixed by the time value associated with simple visual reaction time, and let us assume here a value of 160 msec (shown on the time base as 30 + 100 + 30 = 160 msec). Since Lindsley[19] has estimated that "only about 50 to 60 msec are required for impulses to get to and from the brain in the reaction-time situation," (p. 82) we need to specify at what point in the remaining 100 msec (i.e., 160 msec for RT − 60 msec for transmission = 100 msec for central processing) the SVE component becomes implicated in the processing sequence.

To identify, by means of a time marker, the transition state of a visual input entering the SVE component, a "gate" or "gating mechanism," as is shown in FIGURE 1, is used 100 msec in time after the input has entered the visual cortex, or about 130 msec in time after the input has impinged on the *S*'s retina. This value of about 100 to 130 msec implies that when a string of inputs enters the visual system, each input must pass through a succession of data, or information processing stages (duration about 130 msec) prior to passing through the gate and entering the SVE component of our model. In effect, we are stating quite explicitly that man's visual experience of external events "lags" behind the actual occurrence of these events on the order of about 1/10 of a second.

We have arrived at this 100-to-130-msec value of real-time input processing prior to SVE processing from the sequential blanking and displacement phenomena discussed earlier. Specifically, we have observed for the display sequences shown in TABLE 1, plus many hundreds more that we have examined over the

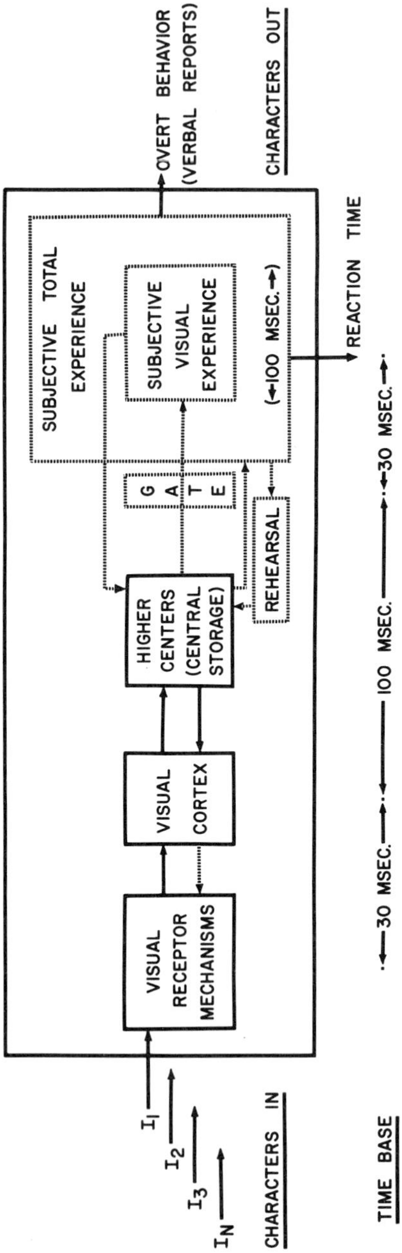

FIGURE 1. Model of visual information processing system.

past three years, that if certain spatio-temporal relationships obtain among a string of inputs, up to 50% of the input string may not be perceived, even with input strings that contain as many as 100 totally discrete inputs (see Reference 25 for an extensive review of such display sequence). Thus, with a string of sequentially displayed inputs, if certain spatio-temporal relationships obtain, the first half or the first 100 to about 130 msec of the displayed inputs may not be perceived. Now, if the first 100 to 130 msec of an input string are lost, it suggests that inputs that are being displayed about 100 msec later in time may prevent the earlier displayed (and blanked) inputs from being perceived. It seems to us that the most plausible mechanism for understanding how "something occurring later in time can prevent one from seeing something that occurred earlier in time" is to postulate that the earlier inputs had not yet reached SVE. Thus, the gate in our model represents a critical temporal stage in the processing of a visual input.

Let us examine more carefully the gating mechanism, which is central to our model. We have introduced a gating mechanism or gate into our model to serve as a time marker for the occurrence of very critical events that occur during the processing of a string of inputs. Let us first examine the case in which the inputs occur in adjacent spatial locations (i.e., sequential blanking and sequential displacement phenomena); we will subsequently discuss the case in which the inputs occur in the same spatial location (i.e., overprinting phenomena), and a special situation, in which blanking and overprinting are combined into a single experimental paradigm. TABLE 2 gives a number of display sequences of varying lengths, in which the numbers give the display order, as in TABLE 1, and underlined numbers represent those display locations in which characters typically are not perceived. First, however, let us indicate, that if display "on" + "off" times sum to appreciably less than 100 msec, all characters are perceived clearly and as occurring simultaneously, while if they sum to appreciably more than 300 msec, all characters are perceived clearly and as occurring sequentially; thus, blanking is maximized at about 200 msec of total display time, independent of sequential input length.

Two very important results emerge, as seen in TABLE 2. First, blanking occurs for inputs which are spatially adjacent to inputs which have occurred about 100 msec earlier in time, either on both sides of the blanked inputs, as in $3\underline{1}4\underline{2}5$, or only on one side, as in $\underline{1}435\underline{2}$. Second, and perhaps of greater importance, it may be noted that for certain mixed content sequences (e.g. – / – /– or / – / – /) with a display order (e.g. 31425) that typically produces blanking, no blanking occurs. Also, with the several 40 "X" sequences shown and in which only 20 "X's"

TABLE 2

SELECTED DISPLAY ORDERS FOR SEVERAL CHARACTER SEQUENCES

	5-Character Sequences			
	C H A I R	/ / / / /	– / – / –	. . . . .
	X X X X X	– – – – –	/ – / – /	! ! ! ! !
Display	1 2 3 4 5	1 2 3 4 5	1 2 3 4 5	1 2 3 4 5
Orders	5 4 3 2 1	5 4 3 2 1	5 4 3 2 1	5 4 3 2 1
	2 4 $\underline{1}$ 3 5	3 $\underline{1}$ 4 $\underline{2}$ 5	3 1 4 2 5	3 $\underline{1}$ 4 $\underline{2}$ 5
	$\underline{1}$ 4 3 5 $\underline{2}$	Display Times:	On time = 20 msec	
	3 $\underline{1}$ 4 $\underline{2}$ 5		Off time = 20 msec	

TABLE 2 (*Cont.*)
40-Character Sequences

X	X	X	X	X	X	X	X	X	X	X	X	X	X	X	X	X	X	X	X	X	X	X	X	X	X	X	X	X	X	X	X	X	X	X	X	X	X	X	X
1	21	2	22	3	23	4	24	5	25	6	26	7	27	8	28	9	29	10	30	11	31	12	32	13	33	14	34	15	35	16	36	17	37	18	38	19	39	20	40
21	1	2	22	23	3	4	24	25	5	6	26	27	7	8	28	29	9	10	30	31	11	12	32	33	13	14	34	35	15	16	36	37	17	18	38	39	19	20	40
21	22	1	2	3	4	23	24	25	26	5	6	7	8	27	28	29	30	9	10	11	12	31	32	33	34	13	14	15	16	35	36	37	38	17	18	19	20	39	40
21	22	1	2	3	4	5	23	24	25	26	27	6	7	8	9	10	28	29	30	31	32	11	12	13	14	15	33	34	35	36	37	16	17	18	19	20	38	39	40
21	22	23	24	25	26	27	1	2	3	4	5	6	7	8	9	10	28	29	30	31	32	33	11	12	13	14	15	16	17	18	19	20	34	35	36	37	38	39	40
21	22	23	24	25	26	27	28	29	30	1	2	3	4	5	6	7	8	9	10	11	12	13	14	15	16	17	18	19	20	31	32	33	34	35	36	37	38	39	40
1	2	3	4	5	6	7	8	9	10	30	11	31	12	32	13	33	14	34	15	35	16	36	17	37	18	38	19	39	20	40	21	22	23	24	25	26	27	28	29

Display times:
On time = 2.5 msec
Off time = 2.5 msec

TABLE 2 (*Cont.*)

100-Character Sequence

(1) A 10 × 10 matrix of (1) all "X's" or all "–s," (2) alternate columns of "X's and "O's" or "–s" and "/s," and (3) the top five rows alternate columns of "–s" and "/s" and bottom five rows all "–s."

1	51	2	52	3	53	4	54	5	55	
6	56	7	57	8	58	9	59	10	60	
11	61	12	62	13	63	14	64	15	65	
16	66	17	67	18	68	19	69	20	70	
21	71	22	72	23	73	24	74	25	75	Display times:
26	76	27	77	28	78	29	79	30	80	On time = 1 msec
31	81	32	82	33	83	34	84	35	85	Off time = 1 msec
36	86	37	87	38	88	39	89	40	90	
41	91	42	92	43	93	44	94	45	95	
46	96	47	97	48	98	49	99	50	100	

Note: "Blanking" as indicated by underlining occurs only for (1) all "X's" or all "–s" and (3) bottom five rows of all "–s," while for (2) alternate columns of "X's" and "O's" or "–s" and "/s" and for (3) top five rows of alternate columns of '–s" and "/s," no "blanking" occurs whatsoever.

are perceived, if the letter "O" is substituted for the letter "X" in each sequence in the blanked locations, all blanking is eliminated, and 20 "X's" interleaved with 20 "O's" are clearly perceived. Again, the 10 × 10 matrix, shown in TABLE 2, shows clearly the modulation of blanking effects by input content or geometry, also as noted in TABLE 2. The results shown in TABLE 2 indicate clearly that spatiotemporal factors give rise to sequential blanking phenomena, but that the blanking effect may be eliminated if certain geometric relationships obtain among the inputs. The 10 × 10 matrix array is particularly revealing in demonstrating the effects of input geometry in that in a single input configuration, the top five rows yield no blanking of alternate columns, where –s and /s interleave, while the bottom five rows yield total blanking of alternate columns, where only –s appears in all ten columns.

What underlying processing mechanisms are responsible for the sequential blanking and displacement effects just outlined? Let us assume that each sequential input, as it enters the visual system, passes through a number of processing stages, perhaps some serially and perhaps some in parallel, finally arriving at SVE, whose function is to provide *S* with a subjective visual experience of external reality. Assume further that the final visual experience is a resultant of certain excitatory and inhibitory processes associated with each input and all other inputs associated "closely" with it, in space and time. The argument that we will now develop depends crucially on the role of inhibitory mechanisms in the visual system, described so elegantly by Ratliff[30] in his recent book on Mach bands, combined with the recent findings of Hubel and Wiesel[13-15] on cat and monkey striate cortex. Hubel and Wiesel[15] state, for example: "From this and previous studies it is clear that any small region of the striate cortex analyses some small part of the visual field in terms of the direction of light-dark contours (in particular, the tangent to the contour lines), a detection of movement of the contours, a registration of the type of contour (light against dark, edge, and the like), and at the hypercomplex level, a detection of any change in direction (curvature) of the contours." (p. 238) This analysis by Hubel and Wiesel suggests a multiplicity of "geometric and brightness analyzers" or processing mechanisms that the visual system brings to bear on each visual input, and we shall take the position that this analysis process requires about 1/10 of a second to be carried out in the human visual system, as we previously indicated, and results in the input entering the SVE component of our model.

Continuing further, we shall assume, based on the findings summarized by Ratliff[30] on lateral inhibition, in particular, and by von Békésy[1] on sensory inhibition, in general, that each input to man's visual system is characterized by a mapping onto the visual cortex, at some level, in which the input itself represents a central excitatory field surrounded by an inhibitory field. Thus, if the excitatory and inhibitory fields of a string of inputs begin to overlap, interactions will develop and sequential blanking and displacement effects may occur.

However, for such sequential blanking and displacement effects actually to occur, at least two conditions must be fulfilled: (1) the inputs must be in close spatial proximity (i.e., within a few degrees of visual angle to one another), and (2) the inputs must be separated in time by about 1/10 of a second. If the two preceding conditions produce sequential blanking and displacement effects, how can we account for the effects of input geometry in modulating or totally eliminating such effects, as shown in TABLE 2? Results that were fully confirmed in two additional studies, in which either five vertical lines[6] or five squares[21] displayed so as to yield sequential blanking effects revealed a systematic decline in blanking effects to zero values, as either the blanked lines were made shorter or longer or the blanked squares were slowly changed into trapezoids.

Since we already know that inhibitory fields operate only over a certain distance in the visual cortex, let us assume that as a result of "geometric analyzers," inputs with different geometric properties are "routed" to different locations in the visual cortex, sufficiently distant from one another so that the inhibitory fields of these later inputs do not interact with the excitatory fields of the earlier inputs arriving in the system. The work of Hubel and Wiesel,[13–15] we believe, provides a sound basis for the above speculations. Geometric analyzers or, more generally, form and contour processing mechanisms, as suggested by Hubel and Wiesel,[15] are characterized by a columnar system for dealing "with multidimensional problems using a two-dimensional surface. In the visual system the two co-ordinates of the visual field are mapped on the two surface co-ordinates; other variables, notably line orientation, eye dominance, possibly movement directionality, are handled by subdividing this surface into overlapping mosaics which are independent." (p. 241–242) If we finally assume that as a result of about the first 100 to 130 msec of input processing, inputs are "routed" to locations within this columnar system, and that if the inputs arrive in the same column, because of sufficient geometric similarities, along dimensions such as, line length or orientation, angle size, degree of curvature, and so on, then these inputs may fall sufficiently close to one another for inhibitory fields to interact and so produce sequential blanking effects. On the other hand, if sufficient geometric differences exist along dimensions, such as line length or orientation, angle size, and others, then these inputs will be "routed" to different columns, and thus may *not* fall sufficiently close to one another for inhibitory fields to interact, and therefore, little if any sequential blanking effects should occur.

Thus, the above formulation provides both a plausible explanation for the effects of input content on sequential blanking effects, but more importantly, provides a powerful experimental paradigm for beginning to establish the invariant dimensions of feature extraction processing and the assessment of the processing rules exercised by the visual system in form and pattern perception.

We will have more to say about this crucial component of pattern perception in our later discussion dealing with the combination of blanking and over-printing paradigms.

With sequential displacement (as demonstrated in TABLE 1 with the word "SOMERSAULT" and the display order 13579246810), we believe, as a first approximation, since the letter "S" displayed second is not blanked but merely spatially displaced to the right of the input letter "R," that this phenomena also results from an inhibitory field effect. However, this type of inhibitory effect is a very unbalanced effect, since the displaced input letter "S," has an input letter "R" to its left that occurs 130 msec later in time, while to its right it has an input letter "A," that occurs only 30 msec later in time. This considerable time imbalance between excitatory and inhibitory field interactions gives rise apparently to a spatial displacement in a direction away from the later occurring field, but much further work is required to understand better why such a time imbalance of excitatory and inhibitory fields should give rise to such spatial displacement effects. We shall refer later to an even more dramatic spatial displacement effect, which unfortunately does not even fit the above rather sparse formulation.

To return again to the critical role played by the gate in our model, in the light of the immediately preceding considerations, a very crucial question arises, namely, "why are the inhibitory mechanisms operative in this gating mechanism exerting effects 100 to 130 msec later in time and not immediately?" We would speculate as follows: For example, with a display sequence of 5 "X's" and a display order such 31425, five "X's" are clearly perceived, if "on" and "off" times are five msec, or less, while blanking, as noted, is maximized for "on" and "off" times of 20 msec. We would assume that the five "X's" are all processed by a letter "X" filter, located somewhere between visual receptor mechanisms and the gate, and which has a limited capacity for resolving both temporal order and spatial location simultaneously at high input rates, such as 5 msec or less for "on" and "off" times, and therefore, codes the message correctly with respect to its occupying five spatial locations, but loses all information concerning temporal ordering. We must also assume that the inhibitory fields associated with the slightly later arriving inputs are not sufficiently strong to inhibit the excitatory fields of the slightly earlier arriving inputs, and so inhibition of inputs at the gate is absent. At the somewhat slower rate of 20 msec, for "on" and "off" times, we enter a highly critical time domain, in which input 1 is just about to enter SVE when input 3 and, shortly thereafter, input 4 arrive in the visual cortex. Since the time separation now is too great for "packaging" or processing all inputs together, temporal ordering becomes more likely. However, the inhibitory fields of the later inputs are now much stronger than the excitatory fields of the earlier inputs, which are slowly decaying with time; thus inhibitory interactions occur at the gate and the excitatory fields associated with the earlier arriving inputs become greatly attenuated by the inhibitory fields associated with the later arriving inputs. This excitatory-inhibitory field interaction produces the sequential blanking and displacement effects, as noted. Of course, if the "on" and "off" times are extended to 40 or 50 msec, then little, if any, interaction occurs between successive excitatory and inhibitory fields, and all inputs pass through the gate and both spatial and temporal ordering is correctly coded, with a resultant verdical and isomorphic match of output to input.

If our above conception of inhibitory fields is meaningful, then with appropriate paradigms, it should be possible to map the shape of such fields within the visual cortex, and we have made a small beginning in this direction.[33] Specifically, we chose for our input a very simple geometric shape, namely, a point source of light, with luminance of each point about 1 ml. Five such point sources were then displayed sequentially in a single horizontal line on the CRT console, with the display order 31425. The *S* sat 36″ from the display. The five points were each .45″ from one another and preliminary pilot work showed that if the separation or distance between each point began to exceed .60″ to .70″, then five points were always clearly perceived, while with the .45″ of separation, only three points were reported as seen, the two end points and the middle point, identical to results shown in TABLE 2 for this display order with "CHAIR" or "XXXXX." The two blanked points were then moved into over 150 different spatial locations in the interspace between the three blanking points, both vertically and horizontally.

The results showed clearly that if the blanked points fell anywhere within a rectangular band about .10″ above and below the horizontal line of the three blanking points or back and forth along this horizontal line, sequential blanking effects were almost 100%. Above and below this rectangular band was a second band extending from about .10″ to about .50″, in which a perception of phi-like movement was reported, with the three blanking points serving as the termini of these movements, and above and below this movement band was a third rectangular band, i.e., above or below .50″, in which all five points were almost always reported as being present. It is our present hypothesis that these rectangular inhibitory and movement-like bands correspond directly to the columnar arrangement of the visual cortex, as suggested by the studies of Hubel and Wiesel,[13–15] and which would result from a series of three overlapping inhibitory circular fields, each associated with one of the three blanking point sources. More importantly, by employing point light sources and different spatial arrangements or input display orders, it should now prove possible to develop systematically a rather fine-grain mapping of excitatory and inhibitory field interactions within the visual cortex by positioning point light sources in a manner somewhat analogous to the positioning of microelectrodes in cat or monkey striate cortex, and assuming that blanking functions in man correspond to frequency of neuron firings in cat and monkey striate cortex.

Since point light sources show the same sequential blanking effects as the more complex letter arrays shown in TABLES 1 and 2, a study was carried out[2] in which the sides of triangles, squares, pentagons, hexagons, and irregular 6- and 12-sided polygons were displayed sequentially. We again found very strong sequential blanking effects, for the first half of the figure, if the whole figure was displayed sequentially, i.e., side after side, within a total display time of about 200 msec. We have tested this finding further by partitioning a Necker Cube into three, six, or 12 sequential "chunks" (i.e., the front face, the four connecting lines to the back face, and the back face, or the six faces, or the 12 edges) and again employing a total display time of 200 msec, with equal time partitioning to display the "chunks" sequentially. Again, *S*'s report as missing, with three "chunks," the first "chunk," and with six and 12 "chunks," the first three and six "chunks," respectively. Thus, one is forced to conclude that even with a geometric structure as complex and ambiguous as a Necker Cube, sequential blanking effects operate almost without exception. In fact, we have as yet found only one condition with closed geometric figures in which blanking effects are somewhat attenuated, namely, if the size of the figure is made quite large, e.g. a 6″ square versus a 2″ square; then the blanking effect is considerably weakened. We would tentatively conclude from this that the larger size figures make it increasingly less probably that the inhibitory fields will spatially overlap the excitatory fields, which leads to the blanking effects.

Before finally completing our discussion of sequential blanking and displacement effects and dealing with overprinting effects, we should like to report on some data just collected that bear directly on additional factors which may modulate sequential blanking effects, beyond the effects of input geometry. As previously indicated in TABLE 1, with the word "SOMERSAULT" and the display order 16273849510, and with the appropriate input display rates (i.e., 10 msec "on" and "off" per letter), *S*'s typically report seeing only the letters "O," "E," "S," "U," and "T." We also had previously used this input display order, but interleaving two different five-letter words, as follows: "BCEAARCRHY."[25] Since, at that time, this was only a very preliminary probe into the effects of word meaning on sequential blanking effects, no firm conclusions were made, although for the four S's who viewed this display, blanking did seem to occur, with the *S*'s reporting only the word "CARRY," the word "BEACH" being blanked. We have had occasion to question this result, based on more recent and extensive findings,[9] and therefore, we have just completed a brief experiment designed specifically to begin to explore this area more carefully.

Some ten *S*'s were given 30 display trials, employing the display order and input rate just discussed. On ten trials, two highly common five-letter words, e.g. "TABLE" and "CHAIR," were interleaved, such as "TCAHBALIER"; on another ten trials, the first five letters displayed did not make a word, such as "MHBOLUXSUE," where only the second five letters displayed form the word "HOUSE," and on the remaining ten trials, ten ten-letter words were employed, such as "SOMERSAULT," "EXPERIMENT," and others.

The results were quite clear. If two five-letter words were interleaved, almost all *S*'s reported both words correctly, i.e., 91% correct reports for the words in which the letters were displayed sixth, seventh, eighth, ninth, and tenth, and 87% correct reports for the words in which the letters were displayed first, second, third, fourth, and fifth. In sharp contrast, when random letters were interleaved with a single five-letter word, the word again was reported with an accuracy of 88%, while the individual letters displayed first, second, third, fourth, and fifth, yielded the following values: 21, 6, 4, 8, and 12%, respectively. With the ten ten-letter words, not one *S* ever reported seeing a single one of the ten-letter words, and the percentage of letters reported correctly were as follows: 18, 84, 2, 78, 4, 71, 3, 72, 11, and 65%.

The implications of these results seem clear. If the first five letters displayed form a word, the inhibitory field effects of the last five letters displayed prove almost totally ineffective in producing sequential blanking effects, while if the first five letters do *not* form a word, whether the second five letters form a word or not, inhibitory effects are very strong and sequential blanking occurs most readily. Thus, it would appear that not only can input content or geometry greatly modulate sequential blanking effects, but also word meaning can produce equally powerful modulating or attenuating effects on sequential blanking. This finding is especially important to the development of our model, since it now appears that as the individual inputs pass through the "visual cortex" and "higher centers" (i.e., central storage) components of our model, not only may input geometry produce different "routes" or "pathways" leading to spatial locations sufficiently different to eliminate inhibitory field interactions, but also word meaning may produce equivalent processings. Since one typically assumes that word recognition and word meaning involve higher centers and central storage mechanisms, our results suggest that such higher centers must be deeply implicated in the processing of visual inputs prior to SVE processing. In sum, the sequential blanking paradigm may allow for a spatial mapping of inputs, in the visual cortex and higher centers, differing not only along geometric dimensions, but also along "meaning" dimensions as well.

Overprinting Effects

In dealing with sequential blanking and displacement effects, we have assumed that the several excitatory fields associated with a string of adjacently located sequential inputs fall within the inhibitory fields of later inputs in the input string, and a complex cascade of excitatory-inhibitory field interactions may result. In dealing with overprinting effects, since the successive inputs are all being displayed in the same general location in space, i.e., in the same cell location on the CRT display surface, the several excitatory fields of the input string are directly superimposed or overlapping one another in space, and we shall assume that the fundamental interaction that now occurs is primarily among the excitatory fields themselves, rather than between the excitatory fields of earlier inputs and the inhibitory fields of later inputs, in the input string. Suppose, for example, we display the letters "A" and "B" simultaneously for 10 msec in the same spatial location on the CRT display surface and ask an *S* to report his visual experience. Since our alpha-numeric characters are made by intensifying the appropriate points in a 5 × 7 matrix of points[24] the simultaneous display of two letters, such as "A" and "B," leads to a visual experience of a "jumble of points of light" and no discernible letter or letters. However, if we display the letters "L" and "T" in a like manner, since the points making up the two letters are not interwoven, almost all *S*'s will accurately report "L" and "T" occurring together, if asked what letters are present.

In four studies[12,16,27,28] we have begun to examine some of the interactions that occur when we display letters on top of letters, digits on top of digits and words on top of words, and to relate these findings to the multiple interactions of successive excitatory fields. Three basic parameters have been systematically varied in one or more of these four studies, i.e., display "on" time per input, display "off" time between inputs or interstimulus interval (ISI), and list length or the number of inputs in the input string.

We have found,[12] for example, that if two sequential letters or three- or five-letter words are displayed one on top of another, percent correct detections increases with both (1) increases in "on" time for a given level of "off" time, and (2) increases in "off" time for a given level of "on" time, with "on" time values of 5, 10, 25, and 50 msec and "off" time values of 1, 10, 25, 50, 75, 100, and 125 msec. Further, and of more concern to our model, "off" time appears to play a more important role than "on" time, for a given total processing time. Thus, comparing an "on + off + on" time combination, such as 25 + 10 + 25 msec, which equals a total processing time period of 60 msec, with an "on + off + on" time combination, such as 5 + 50 + 5 msec, which also equals a total processing time period of 60 msec, percent correct detections is only 57% on the average with 10 msec of "off" time, while it jumps to 85% on the average with 50 msec of "off" time. We would interpret this finding to mean that for a given total processing time period, increases in "off" time provides for more time between the excitatory fields associated with each input, and therefore, less interaction between the successive excitatory fields should result, with a concomitant increase in detections, as was found. It should be noted, however, that this relationship between "on" and "off" times has a limiting value, and work is currently in progress on this problem.

Another, and perhaps more intriguing finding of our work on overprinting may be found in the results shown in TABLE 3. These results, obtained from two previous studies,[16,27] show percent correct detections for varying length digit strings (in which digit "on" time was 10 msec) as a function of different ISI values for all serial positions of the digit string. First, one may observe in TABLE 3 that only with an ISI value of 300 msec do percent correct detections begin to approach 100% for all length strings. That is, ISI values less than 300 msec produce increasing decrements in detection performance as list length increases, and this is true for word strings as well.[3,28] If only two inputs are employed, however, there is no hint whatsoever that interactions among inputs might be extended over a time period as long as 300 msec. Further, the serial position analysis shown in TABLE 3 strongly suggests that the interactions between successive inputs in the longer length strings at the shorter ISI values are not simple linear interactions, since marked U-shaped serial position curves are found, rather than a general depression of detection performance at all serial positions. Thus, it would appear that multiple interacting excitatory fields summate in complicated nonlinear ways, and further work is clearly required to formalize and conceptualize these nonlinear interactions more effectively. Finally, the finding that interaction effects seem to be eliminated from the longer length strings only when an ISI value of 300 msec is reached suggests the following formulation concerning the flow of inputs through the visual system. Namely, the total input processing for a short duration input (such as 10 msec "on" time) requires about 300 msec, divided approximately into 100 to 130 msec of processing prior to SVE, about 100 msec within SVE, and about 100 msec for trace consolidation in central storage.[27,28] In effect, we are suggesting a continuous dynamic processing of a visual input for at least 300 msec after it enters the visual system, in which many and varied mechanisms are brought to bear, the net result of which allows *S* to report or respond in some appropriate fashion as to the nature of the input, and any disruption of input processing during this first 300 msec can produce one or more of the types of spatio-temporal interactions we have been considering.

Sequential Blanking and Overprinting Combined

In the experimental paradigm that we shall now discuss,[22] we believe a very powerful technique for assessing certain critical problem areas in pattern, contour, or form perception has evolved. Specifically, the display order 31425 previously discussed and shown in TABLE 2 as yielding strong sequential blanking effects for

TABLE 3

PERCENT CORRECT DETECTIONS FOR SERIAL POSITION ANALYSIS (N = 10)

	2 Digit String		3 Digit String			4 Digit String				5 Digit String				
ISI (msec)	1	2	1	2	3	1	2	3	4	1	2	3	4	5
20	58	50	34	22	14	32	4	4	60	30	2	4	8	44
40	72	84	66	14	68	72	8	16	58	60	2	2	10	72
60	86	98	66	36	90	70	22	12	78	70	16	0	16	68
80	88	92	62	44	80	76	42	38	72	74	18	12	24	74
100	85	90	74	62	94	76	44	42	90	74	36	18	24	70
300	100	100	98	98	98	96	92	92	96	100	98	94	92	90

the inputs displayed first and second, was chosen as the blanking pattern to combine with the overprinting paradigm. However, before combining blanking and overprinting, some 60 letter pairs, such as, "S" and "N," "G" and "P," "B" and "X," and so on, were displayed using the overprinting paradigm alone, to a small sample of *S*'s (N = 4) four times each in a random order for a total of 240 trials. The "on + off + on" time combination for each letter pair was 20 msec "on" + 50 μsec "off" + 20 msec "on." As might be expected with such "on-off" times, percent correct letter detections was quite low and the ten pairs of 60 showing the lowest detection values were selected for the combined blanking-overprinting paradigm.

For these ten lowest pairs, the average percent correct detections of letters was only 9.5%. For each of these ten pairs two basic blanking patterns were generated. For example, the letter pair "S" and "N" yielded the two patterns shown in TABLE 4. In TABLE 4, the display order is shown with the underlined numbers representing the input locations displayed first and second, and which are typically blanked with this display order, if all inputs are the same. Also, it may be seen that in the input locations displayed first and second "N" and "S" have been typed one above the other to indicate overprinting of "N" and "S" in these display locations. In the left hand array, the "S" is displayed before the "N" and in the right hand array the "N" is displayed before the "S." Five ISI values were selected for the separation time of the two overprinted inputs, namely, 50 μsec, 1 msec, 10 msec, 50 msec, and 100 msec, while "on" and "off" times for the remaining five identical letters, i.e., "N's" in the left-hand array and "S's" in the right hand array, were 20 msec "on" and 20 msec "off." With ten different letter pairs each generating two basic displays, like those shown in TABLE 4, and with five different ISI values for the overprinted inputs, each of the ten *S*'s employed in the study received a total of 100 trials. Since we know that (1) five identical letters will produce strong sequential blanking effects and (2) in the blanked locations there are two overprinted inputs separated from each other in time by varying ISI values, the question is raised regarding how the visual system will process such a sequential input stream, having both features of blanking and overprinting combined. For example, with an ISI value of 50 μsec, we know percent correct letter detections is close to zero for the pure overprinting case. Now, with the sequential blanking pattern added to the processing sequence, as in the left hand array of TABLE 4, will the second and fourth display locations be "cleared" of the identical letter, i.e., "N," and thus allow the "S" to be detected?

The percent correct detections for the letter displayed first in the overprinted locations were 37, 43, 56, 92, and 93% for ISI values of 50 μsec, 1 msec, 10 msec, 50 msec, and 100 msec, respectively. Thus, the results clearly demonstrate that a fourfold increase in percent correct detections, i.e., from 9.5%, with overprinting alone to 37% with a blanking pattern added, is possible with only a 50 μsec ISI value. These results represent a far higher degree of temporal resolving power than is typically attributed to the visual system.[4] More importantly, as an

TABLE 4

TYPICAL BLANKING AND OVERPRINTING DISPLAY PATTERN

Display		S		S				N		N	
Characters	N	N	N	N	N		S	S	S	S	S
						or					
Display Order	3	$\underline{1}$	4	$\underline{2}$	5		3	$\underline{1}$	4	$\underline{2}$	5

experimental paradigm for studying pattern perception, we may now begin to make a rather fine-grained analysis of feature extraction in the visual system. By systematically varying the input geometry of the two overprinted inputs and their relationship to the input geometry of the blanking inputs, as well as the ISI values separating the two overprinted inputs, we should be able to identify at least some of the processing and coding routines employed by the visual system in pattern perception. For example, suppose in TABLE 4, we reverse the orders in which we display the two overprinted inputs, and again vary ISI values between these two inputs. How will these changes affect percent correct detections? Or suppose we employ letters, such as "L" and "T," which do not yield poor detection scores when overprinted, and again follow these overprinted inputs with a blanking pattern of "L's" or "T's." How will these types of changes affect percent correct detections? Answers to such questions raised by a blanking-overprinting paradigm should help in unraveling the coding mechanisms employed by the visual system in pattern perception.

Finally, and very briefly, we should like to discuss the implications of the above findings for our model. The results obtained would suggest that while the excitatory fields of the two overprinted inputs, particularly at an ISI value of only 50 μsec, must be coded together in the SVE component of our model, since they are experienced together as a composite jumble of points (if no blanking inputs are present), they must also be coded separately at least 37% of the time at some point prior to SVE, since the inhibitory fields of the blanking inputs operate selectively 37% of the time to blank only one of the two inputs present in the blanked location. It is our hope that a thorough exploitation of the blanking-overprinting paradigm should appreciably extend the range of our model into the area of pattern and form perception.

Continuously Cycling Displays

In all of the studies discussed so far, we have employed display sequences that represent "discrete" sequential input strings, i.e., input strings that are displayed once, and *S* is then asked to report on his visual experience. We should now like to consider very briefly the case of continuously cycling input strings, i.e., input strings that are not displayed just once, but continue to cycle, with the intercycle interval (ICI) time equal to the ISI time of the input string. We will discuss only one particular display order with a string of 20 inputs to demonstrate some of the very dramatic effects and changes that occur with this display order when input content is changed. TABLE 5 gives the several different contents examined and the display order used, as well as the "on," "off," and ICI times needed to produce the effects we shall now describe. For the line of 20 "O's," all *S*'s report seeing one of two organizations, which reverse back and forth, as in Necker Cube reversals. In one organization, one "sees" a line of 20 "O's" with a slight flicker noticeable, which may suddenly change to a second organization of from five to six "O's" spaced equally apart across the width of the display surface (about 10″), and moving from left to right, just as "ducks in a shooting gallery." If for the 20 "O's," we substitute any one of the other content lines shown in TABLE 5, all *S*'s again report seeing all 20 characters with a slight flicker, or a sudden change to the "ducks in the shooting gallery" type of movement, but with the different content inputs that are moving from left to right rather unbelievably all occupying the identical spatial location. Even the four different content input array "O–/!" takes on this form, so that it appears as if the letter "O" had a dash, a slash, and an exclamation point inside it. The dash and exclamation point

TABLE 5

INPUT DISPLAY ORDER AND VARIOUS CONTENTS FOR A CONTINUOUSLY CYCLING DISPLAY
("ON" TIME = 5 MSEC, "OFF" TIME = 5 MSEC, ICI = 5 MSEC)

Display Order	1	5	9	13	17	2	6	10	14	18	3	7	11	15	19	4	8	12	16	20
	O	O	O	O	O	O	O	O	O	O	O	O	O	O	O	O	O	O	O	O
	O	-	O	-	O	-	O	-	O	-	O	-	O	-	O	-	O	-	O	-
Display Characters	O	-	/	O	-	/	O	-	/	O	-	/	O	-	/	O	-	/	O	-
	O	-	/	!	O	-	/	!	O	-	/	!	O	-	/	!	O	-	/	!
	-	!	-	!	-	!	-	!	-	!	-	!	-	!	-	!	-	!	-	!

alone, i.e., the last content line in TABLE 5, appears like a plus sign moving across the display surface. At the moment, we will not even attempt to explain this extreme type of spatial displacement and movement effect, but merely note that very complicated spatio-temporal organizational codings of the input string are obviously taking place, that such codings because of the display rates employed would involve highly complex excitatory and inhibitory field interactions, and that these interactions may suddenly change, since the display is perceived at any given time in one of two possible organizations.

A Neglected Display Parameter and Overview

Up to this point in our presentation we have enumerated some six display parameters that may influence the visual information processing of a sequential input string, namely, (1) the number of inputs, (2) the input display order, (3) the input display rate, (4) the input content or geometry, (5) the input spacing, and (6) the input size. We have neglected to mention one final parameter of critical importance, namely, display input intensity or luminance, since, until very recently, we have not been able to vary this parameter independently, but were forced to employ, because of display hardware limitations, essentially equal luminance values for all inputs in our input strings. With display hardware modifications just implemented, we can now begin to vary individual input luminance and will no longer be forced to display inputs all at the same luminance level.

In preliminary pilot work, it is already very clear that sequential blanking effects can be totally eliminated, either by increasing the luminance of the blanked inputs or by decreasing the luminance of the blanking inputs. Obviously, input luminance must now be incorporated into our model, in such a way that the relative strengths of excitatory and inhibitory fields may be directly related to this display parameter. With the added capability of varying input luminance, it would appear that we have exhausted the relevant display parameters that any visual information processing model must be able to conceptualize.

References

1. Békésy, G. von. 1967. Sensory Inhibition. Princeton University Press. Princeton, N. J.
2. Bell, A., R. G. Forster, F. J. Finnegan, M. Katz, J. I. LaSusa & M. S. Mayzner. 1969. Sequential blanking and visual form perception. Psychon. Sci. **15**: 103–104.
3. Bloom, R. F. 1969. Indirect Measurement of the Consolidation Time Required for Visual Perception. Doctoral dissertation, New York University. New York, N. Y.
4. Boynton, R. M. 1962. Spatial vision. Ann. Rev. Psychol. **13**: 171–200.
5. Broadbent, D. E. 1958. Perception and Communication. Pergamon. New York, N. Y.
6. Buchsbaum, W. H. & M. S. Mayzner. 1969. The effects of line length on sequential blanking. Psychon. Sci. **15**: 111–112.
7. DeValois, R. L. 1966. Neural processing of visual information. *In* Frontiers in Physiological Psychology. R. W. Russel, Ed. : 51–91. Academic Press. New York, N. Y.
8. Efron, R. 1967. The duration of the present. Ann. N. Y. Acad. Sci. **138**(2): 713–729.
9. Engelberg, A. A. 1969. The Inhibition-disinhibition Cycle for the Case of Recurrent Metacontrast. Doctoral dissertation. New York University. New York, N. Y.
10. Fraisse, P. 1963. The Psychology of Time. Harper and Row. New York, N. Y.
11. Graham, C. H., Ed. 1965. Vision and Visual Perception. Wiley. New York, N. Y.
12. Greenberg, M., M. S. Helfer & M. S. Mayzner. 1968. Information processing of letter and word pairs as a function of on and off times. Percept. & Psychophys. **4**: 350–360.
13. Hubel, D. H. & T. N. Wiesel. 1959. Receptive fields of single neurones in the cat's striate cortex. J. Physiol. **148**: 574–596.
14. Hubel, D. H. & T. N. Wiesel. 1962. Receptive fields, binocular interaction, and functional architecture in the cat's visual cortex. J. Physiol. **160**: 106–123.

15. Hubel, D. H. & T. N. Wiesel. 1968. Receptive fields and functional architecture of monkey striate cortex. J. Physiol. **195:** 215–243.
16. Katz, M., K. M. Schoenberg & M. S. Mayzner. 1970. Visual information processing of sequentially presented inputs: II. Effects of list length and interstimulus interval values on sub-span storage and retrieval mechanisms. Percept. & Psychophys. In press.
17. Kahneman, D. 1968. Method, findings, and theory in studies of visual masking. Psychol. Bull. **70:** 404–425.
18. Le Grand, Y. 1968. Light, Colour and Vision. Chapman and Hall. London, England.
19. Lindsley, D. B. 1957. Psychophysiology and motivation. *In* Nebraska Symposium on Motivation. M. R. Jones, Ed. : 44–105. University of Nebraska Press. Lincoln, Nebraska.
20. Mayzner, M. S. 1968. The research potential of a computer-based cathode-ray tube display system. Behavior Res. Meth. & Instru. **1:** 41–43.
21. Mayzner, M. S. & M. E. Tresselt. 1969a. Sequential blanking: A function of geometric analyzers in the human visual system. Psychon. Sci. **17:** 77–78.
22. Mayzner, M. S. & M. E. Tresselt. 1969b. A study of sequential blanking and overprinting combined. In preparation.
23. Mayzner, M. S., M. E. Tresselt & A. Cohen. 1966. Preliminary findings on some effects of very fast sequential input rates on perception. Psychon. Sci. **6:** 513–514.
24. Mayzer, M. S., M. E. Tresselt & M. S. Helfer. 1967a. A research strategy for studying certain effects of very fast sequential input rates on the visual system. Psychon. Monogr. Suppl. **2**(5)**:** 73–81.
25. Mayzner, M. S., M. E. Tresselt & M. S. Helfer. 1967b. A provisional model of visual information processing with sequential inputs. Psychon. Monogr. Suppl. **2**(7)**:** 91–108.
26. Mayzner, M. S., M. E. Tresselt, A. J. Adrignolo & A. Cohen. 1967. Further preliminary findings on some effects of very fast sequential input rates on perception. Psychon. Sci. **7:** 281–282.
27. Mayzner, M. E., M. E. Tresselt, J. Checkes & H. A. Hoenig. 1970. Visual information processing of sequentially presented inputs: III. Further effects of list length and interstimulus interval values on sub-span storage and retrieval mechanisms. Percept. Psychophys. In press.
28. Mayzner, M. E., M. E. Tresselt, N. Tabenkin, R. Didner & M. S. Helfer. 1969. Visual information precessing of sequentially presented inputs: I. Effects of input timing on sub-span storage and retrieval mechanisms. Percept. & Psychophys. **5:** 297–302.
29. Pieron, H. 1925. Recherches expérimentales sur la marge de variation du temps de latence de la sensation lumineuse (par une méthode de masquage). Ann. Psychol. **26:** 1–30.
30. Ratliff, F. 1965. Mach Bands: Quantitative Studies on Neural Networks in the Retina. Holden Day. San Francisco, California.
31. Rosenblith, W. A., Ed. 1961. Sensory Communication. Wiley. New York, N. Y.
32. Schlosberg, H. 1965. Time relations in serial visual perception. Canad. Psychol. **6a:** 161-172.
33. Schoenberg, K. M., M. Katz & M. S. Mayzner. 1969. The shape of inhibitory fields in the human visual system. In preparation.
34. Stigler, R. 1910. Chronophotische Studien über den Ungebungskontrust. Pflüg. Arch. ges. Physiol. **134:** 365-435.
35. Tresselt, M. E. & M. S. Mayzner. 1969. Estimates of "SVE" processing time. Psychon. Sci. **16:** 103–104.
36. White, C. T. 1963. Temporal numerosity and the psychological unit of duration. Psychol. Monogr. **77**(12)**:** 1–37.
37. Woodworth, R. S. & H. Schlosberg. 1954. Experimental Psychology. Henry Holt. New York, N. Y.

COMPLEXITY AND PREFERENCE IN ANIMALS AND MEN*

Edward L. Walker, Ph.D.†
University of Michigan, Ann Arbor, Mich.

Complexity and preference are terms that are relevant to a theory of behavior I presented at the Nebraska Symposium on Motivation several years ago.[7] The research effort I wish to discuss is based on that theoretical statement. The theory differs very little from an earlier theory published by Dember and Earl (see Dember[2]) and it incorporates concepts developed by Berlyne.[1]

The theory contains a small number of terms or concepts and hypotheses which I should like to review briefly in order to make it possible to use them discriminatively in discussing the research. The terms are: *Psychological Event, Stimulus Complexity, Psychological Complexity* and *Optimal Complexity*. From these is developed a theory of *Preference* or choice among psychological events. A hypothesis concerning expected changes in optimal complexity with experience produces an expected set of *Changes in Complexity and Preference with Experience*. This much is relevant to the experiments to be discussed here. An additional concept, arousal, is in the theory but not germane to these experiments and will not be discussed further.

Psychological Event. This is a term I have used to identify a central unit of activity. A psychological event may be initiated by an external stimulus, but many psychological events have the appearance of spontaneity. A response may result from a psychological event, but many psychological events occur without a visible product. A psychological event may have a conscious representation and, thus, the character of perception, but there are circumstances under which psychological events occur without conscious awareness. Thus the need for such a concept arises from the limitations imposed by the concepts of stimulus, response, perception, and cognition, any or all of which may reflect a psychological event, but none of which is identical.

Stimulus Complexity. This term refers to the complexity of the distal stimulus. The essential characteristic of *stimulus* complexity—as distinguished from *psychological* complexity—is that it should be possible to assign a number to a stimulus that represents its complexity and that this value should remain fixed. Often this appears to be no problem, but I believe appearances to be deceiving. With certain kinds of stimulus materials, one can perform a counting operation. One can have stimuli that vary in the number of dots, or polygons that vary in the number of sides. On *a priori* grounds, it seems reasonable that a card with 50 dots is a more complex stimulus than a card with five, or that a polygon with 20 sides is more complex than a polygon with four sides. Yet, if we subject a set of such materials to psychological scaling procedures, it is very unlikely that there will be perfect agreement between our numerical count and the results of the scaling. One is then tempted to undertake to resolve the discrepancies in terms of factors that were not included in the count—configurational or pattern factors. Alternatively, one can choose one of the two values, the numerical count or the results of psychological scaling, and choose to ignore the other. The question then becomes, which does one choose?

I think there is no question that the choice must be the psychologically derived

* The work reported in this paper was supported by grant no. HD 00904 from the United States Public Health Service.

† The author is supported by a research career award, K6–MH–21, 868.

scale. There are two basic reasons. Many important stimuli are not subject to a counting procedure. If I choose to work with abstract paintings as stimuli, there is no simple counting procedure available that yields complexity values having face validity. Even when one can count some aspect of a stimulus set and even when there is a discrepancy between the ordering on the basis of the count and the ordering on the basis of a psychological scaling technique, it is the latter ordering that is likely to be functional in psychological studies.

In a very fundamental way, all quantification, including counting, is a psychological scaling procedure. One's choice, then, should be a psychological scaling procedure that is applicable to all stimuli. It then becomes clear that to achieve a set of complexity values that can be assigned to stimuli and that do not change—thus creating the illusion that they belong to the stimuli and not to the observer—it is necessary to assign permanent complexity values in terms of mean values for a standard population under standard conditions. This, then, is the definition of *stimulus* complexity: mean ratings of a reference population under reference conditions.

Psychological Complexity. Psychological complexity is a characteristic of a psychological event. When a psychological event is initiated by a stimulus, psychological complexity is the result of an interaction between the single individual and the distal stimulus. Thus one would expect that same stimulus to result in different psychological complexity values in two different individuals or in the same individual at different times.

Optimal Complexity. In theory, optimal complexity is that degree of psychological complexity that the organism will seek to maintain. For any array of stimuli, the organism will order the stimuli from least to most complex, and the organism can be considered to occupy a position on that scale, his optimal complexity level. The organism will prefer stimuli near his optimum rather than stimuli farther away.

Preference. The concept of preference is derived directly from the concept of optimal complexity. It is hypothesized that if an organism is asked to choose which of two stimuli he prefers, he will choose that stimulus that is closer to his optimal complexity level. In human subjects, one can ask for a verbal judgment. In animals, one can determine with which of two or more stimuli an animal chooses to interact.

Changes in Complexity and Preference with Experience. The original Dember and Earl theory[2], as well as my own, postulates that the position the organism occupies on a complexity scale will change with continued experience with the items on the scale, and both predict that the change will be upward toward more complex stimuli. Thus, preferences for musical compositions tend to progress from a liking for simple melodies to a liking for more complex ones, then possibly to classical music, and within classical through a nearly predictable sequence of composers to arrive finally at modern atonal and computer-generated compositions. The progression over a long time span is clearly from the simple to the complex.

Two effects of exposure require some additional specification. There is a short-term satiation effect of exposure. During a continuous period of exposure, the complexity of a stimulus will undergo reduction. This satiation effect is in part temporary and subject to recovery in the period after exposure. However, recovery is not complete, and the long-term progression to a preference for more and more complex stimuli is the result of the accumulation of these small permanent changes.

A second effect of exposure is the generalization of change. In the original Dember and Earl theory it was assumed that (in my terms) the psychological complexities of the items on the scale maintained their relative positions during change produced by an exposure to a single stimulus. Thus, it is implied that generalization was complete. In my own statement of 1964, I operated under the assumption that the items on the scale were independent in the sense that a change in one stimulus produced through interaction with it did not affect the complexity of other stimuli on the scale. Both positions lead to logical difficulties and to a failure to handle much of the sequential choice data. It is probably necessary, therefore, to assume that the effects of exposure to one stimulus are generalized to other stimuli in proportion to distances on the complexity scale.

Two sets of experiments will be discussed. The first set was carried out with human subjects and the second with animals. They will be discussed separately because the special characteristics of the two species (humans and rats) permitted the study of different but related problems.

Stimulus Complexity and Preference in Human Subjects‡

Most of the work that has been done by others in efforts to investigate stimulus preference and complexity has involved either one of two approaches to the selection of stimulus materials. One approach is to select stimulus materials that differ in complexity on the basis of a simple kind of face validity. This approach is handicapped because one cannot plot preference against such nonmetricized stimuli. The second common approach is to generate a set of stimuli with a known physical or quantitative dimensionality.

An alternative approach is to select sets of psychologically interesting stimuli and to subject them to one or more of the psychological scaling techniques. The result might be a set of materials of much more interest than any previously available and a set of materials for which there might be meaningful quantitative dimensions.

In the studies to be discussed in this section, there are generally three aims:

1. To develop sets of visual stimuli with established complexity values based on psychological scaling techniques.
2. To develop methodology for employing these stimuli with human subjects.
3. To investigate the relation of complexity and preference.

The stimuli employed in these studies were derived from four sources:

1. *Tartan Patterns.* A number of tartan patterns were photographed in black and white to serve as stimuli. These had several virtues as stimuli, but one of the most important was that the number of squares in the pattern gave a physical measure of complexity. It was thus possible to check psychological scaling techniques with a physical scale with this one set of stimuli.
2. *Stage Set Designs.* A number of drawings of stage set designs were photographed for use as stimuli. They had the virtue of representing well-established styles in set design that differ in apparent complexity.
3. *Black and White Graphics.* A large set of black and white graphics, all of which were highly representational and symbolic and done by well known artists, was also selected. The graphics had the advantage of being well known to individuals who had studied art, but which were not well known to most individuals.
4. *Modern Art.* A large set of modern paintings was selected. They were chosen

‡ A number of people worked on the stimulus complexity and preference studies from time to time. Much of the work was done by F. Joseph Mortenson, Howard Gadlin, Kathy Nagy, Daneen Hart, and Rivka Fine.

so that they contained no symbolic material and were generally not identifiable in origin. They are colored prints.

All sets of stimulus materials were either chosen in their original form or photographed and reduced to four-by-six-inch pictures. Each was then given a randomly selected code number that was placed on the back. Finally, each was encased with plastic contact acetate to preserve the original quality during handling.

Tartan Patterns

The tartan patterns used in these studies were taken from a volume by Innes.[4] From a larger list, the patterns listed in TABLE 1 were selected and tested. As can be seen in the Table, the number of squares in the sample photographed varied from 91 to 2,680.

In the first study, subjects were asked to rate each of the 21 tartan patterns from simple to complex. They were to use a scale of 1 to 100, with 1 representing the least complex and 100, the most complex. They were then asked to rate each with respect to how much they liked the pattern. Again they were to use a scale ranging from 1 to 100, with 1 representing the least liked, and 100 the most liked, pattern.

The ratings of complexity are compared to the physical properties of the tartan patterns in FIGURE 1. The number of squares is plotted on a log scale as an approximation of the psychophysical function that is probably involved in judging differences in number of squares. The physical scale and the psychological scale are in fairly good agreement in the Figure. Since there are other possibly physical dimensions in the stimuli, such as grey-scale and relative proportions, this level of agreement seems satisfactory. In fact, it seems possible that the psychological scale might come closer to representing complexity than does the physical scale.

TABLE 1

TARTAN PATTERNS BY NAME AND PHYSICAL CHARACTERISTICS

Code Number	Tartan	Number of Rectangles	Number of Rectangles in a Set
1	Royal Stewart	1,375	625
2	Forbes	759	841
3	MacArthur	187	81
4	Skene	1,452	169
5	Brodie	102	121
6	Anderson	2,574	1,326
7	MacDonell of Glengarry	2,109	625
8	MacKay	247	121
9	MacAulay	165	110
10	Kerr	1,760	361
11	Carnegie	999	625
12	Ramsey	375	121
13	Keith	247	81
14	Sutherland	984	529
15	MacDonald of Sleat	273	49
16	Wallace	165	49
17	MacDonald of Clanranald	1,718	625
18	Fraser	247	121
19	Urquart	1,891	729
20	Montgomerie	91	49
21	Maclachlan	405	121

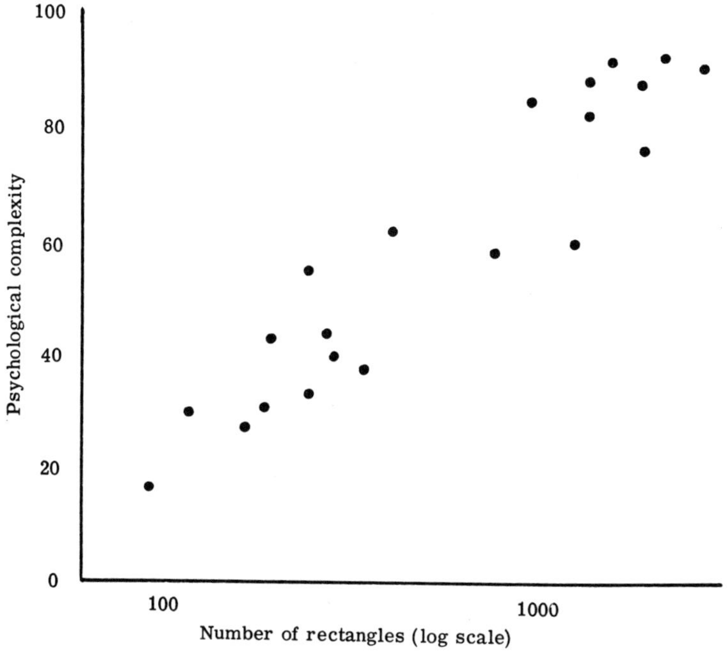

FIGURE 1. Physical versus psychological scales of complexity in Tartan patterns.

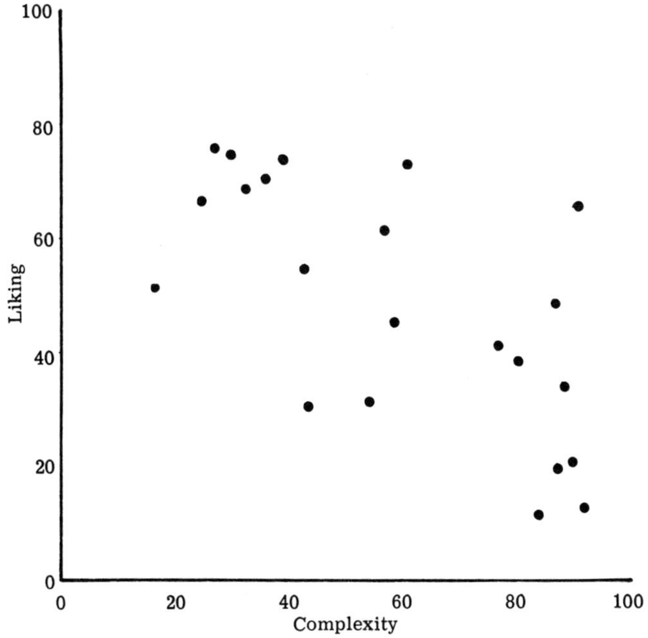

FIGURE 2. Complexity and liking for Tartan patterns.

The relation of the psychological scale of complexity and a similar psychological scale of liking is shown in FIGURE 2. There is an obvious relation between the two measures, with the subjects expressing a greater liking for the simple tartan patterns.

As part of the same study, the subjects were asked to make a second evaluation of the extent to which they liked the tartan patterns. In this case, the patterns were offered in pairs. Subjects were asked to assign a value to the difference in their liking for the two. If the difference in liking was maximum, a value of 10 was to be assigned. If it was minimum, a value of one was to be assigned. Such data can be computer-analyzed, using the Shepard-Kruskal technique.

There are two major advantages to the Shepard-Kruskal scaling and scaling analysis technique. Data collected in this way can be analyzed for any number of dimensions. If a variable such as complexity, liking, or preference is actually multidimensional, the Shepard-Kruskal technique could potentially reveal the fact. The second advantage is that the data collected from a single subject can be subjected to multidimensional analysis. A disadvantage is that a one-dimensional solution is not necessarily the "best" solution. The computer program simply projects a line through the multidimensional space from an arbitrary starting point. It is the best line from that point but not necessarily the best starting point. It is often therefore necessary to ask the computer for an n-dimensional solution and try to match each solution to some criterion. A second disadvantage of the analysis technique is that there are no internal criteria for determining how many dimensions are meaningful. For these reasons, we asked the computer for ten different analyses, specifying numbers of dimensions from 1 to 10 in each case (thus, 55 for each subject). The data from each individual and the group were analyzed separately.

After the subjects had finished their ratings of how well they liked the patterns, they were asked for extensive explanations of the reasons for their liking of a given pattern. Many hours were spent in an effort to match individual Shepard-

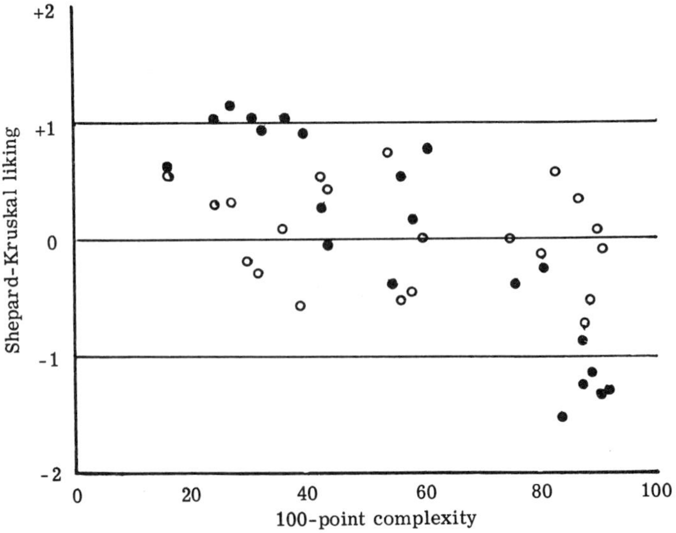

FIGURE 3. Shepard-Kruskal liking dimensions and complexity.

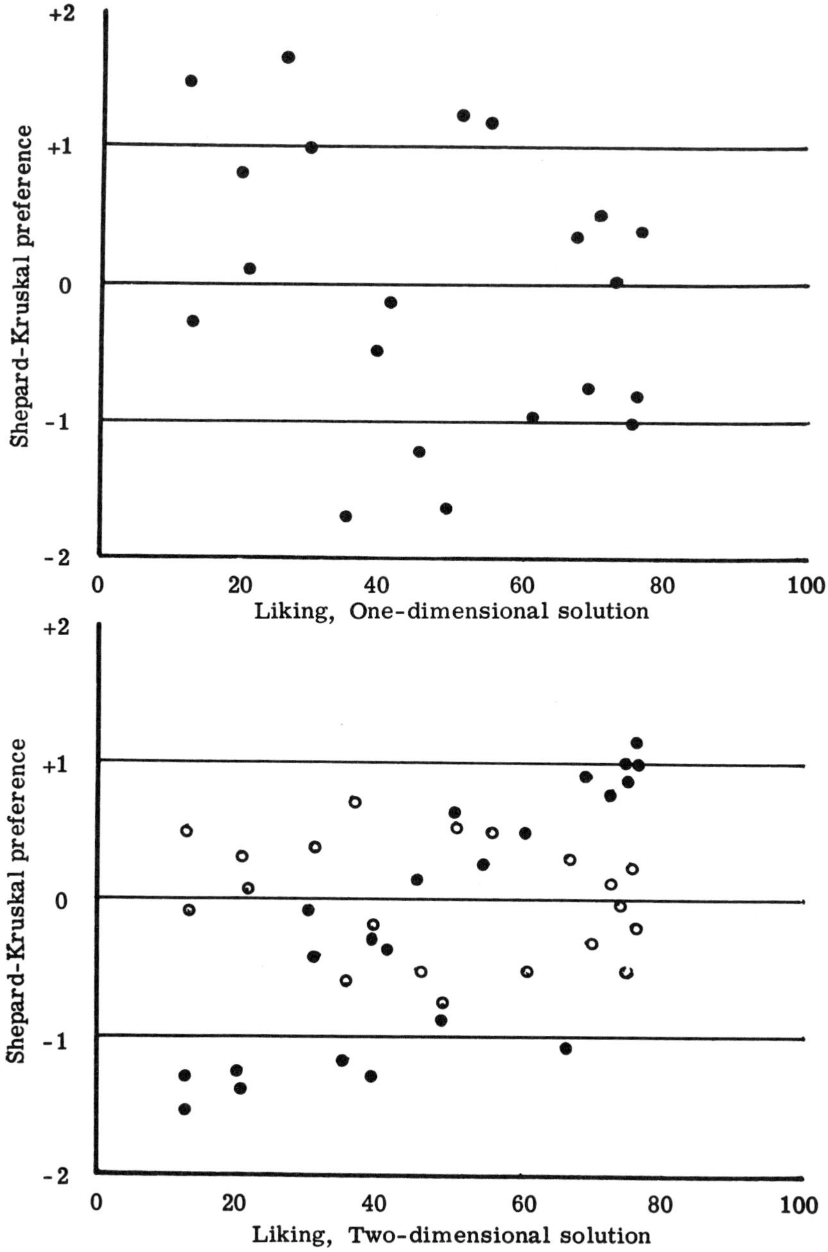

FIGURE 4. Comparison of two scaling procedures.

Kruskal dimensions with the verbal protocols, but the effort was fruitless. Liking seemed to be a single dimension, and elaboration of the basis for liking did not improve understanding of the dimension.

FIGURE 3 is a sample of the Shepard-Kruskal analysis. In this Figure, a two-dimensional solution for liking is plotted against the complexity ratings. The first dimension shows little or no relationship between the two variables. The second dimension shows a clear relationship very similar to that shown in FIGURE 2.

FIGURE 4 is an effort to determine the relationship between the liking scale derived from the simple rating on a 100-point scale and the Shepard-Kruskal analysis of preference. The one-dimensional Shepard-Kruskal solution yields no relationship. When the two dimensions of a two-dimensional solution are plotted, the first dimension shows little or no relationship, while the second dimension shows a rather high correlation.

One further study was carried out with the tartan patterns that was methodological in character. We wished to know what effect the range of stimuli had on ratings of complexity. To determine this, arrangements were made to have subjects rate ten tartan patterns representing the simpler designs, rate ten representing the more complex designs, and rate ten representing the whole range.

The subjects were 15 males and 15 females of college age. They were divided into three groups of ten S's each.

Three sets of stimuli were made up from the tartan patterns that had been rated for complexity in earlier studies. The high complexity set included those rated 1, 2, 3, 4, 6, 7, 8, 9, 10, and 12. The low complexity set included those rated 11, 13, 14, 15, 16, 17, 18, 19, 20, and 21. The full range set included those rated 1, 3, 6, 8, 11, 12, 15, 17, 19 and 21.

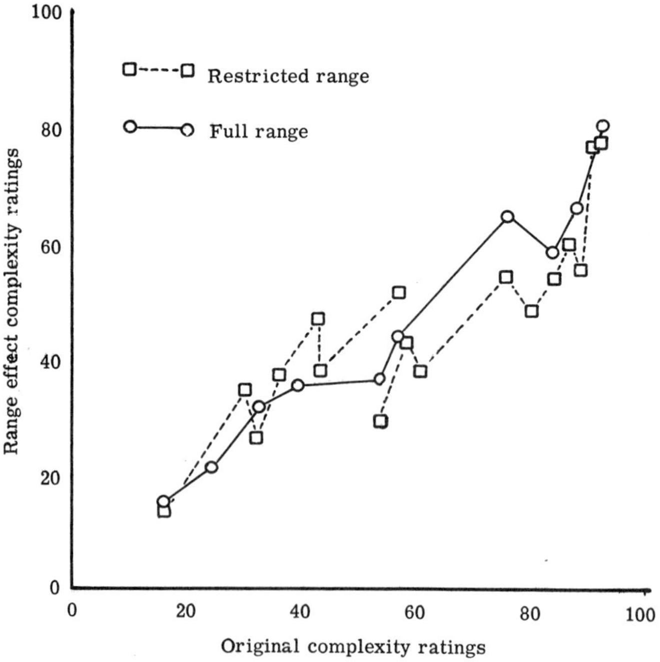

FIGURE 5. Complexity ratings as a function of range of stimuli.

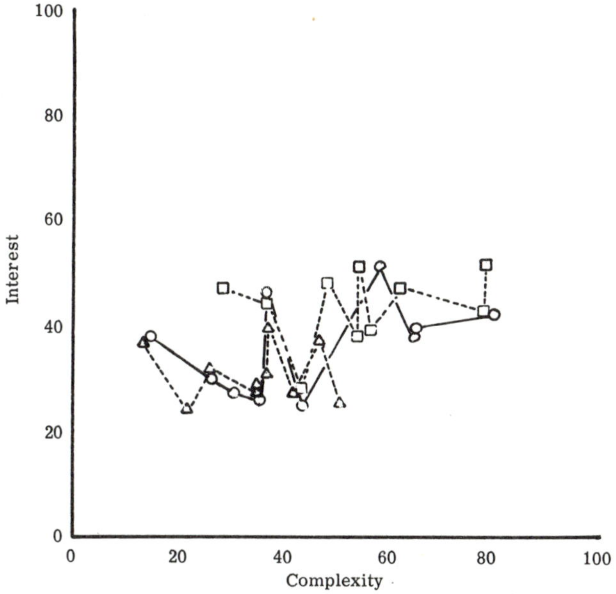

FIGURE 6. Complexity and "interestingness."

Each group rated all three sets. One group rated the low set, then the high, and then the full range set. Another group rated the high, then the low, and then the full range set. The third group rated the full set first and was then split, with half of the S's rating the low complexity set first and the other half, the high complexity set first. This arrangement comes pretty close to counterbalancing order of presentation. Tests for order effect revealed that there was no systematic order effect, and order was therefore ignored in further analysis.

FIGURE 5 is a plot of the results of the three sets of ratings. It is apparent that when subjects rate a restricted range of stimuli, they tend to use more of the range than they do when rating a wider range. Thus the middle range stimuli were rated as more complex when in a set of low complexity and less complex when in a set of higher complexity.

FIGURE 6 is a plot of the second result of this study. In addition to the complexity ratings, the subjects were asked to rate each pattern for "interestingness." Subjects showed very little consistency in their ratings of this variable. What little there is shows the more complex patterns rated as being more interesting. Since earlier subjects had expressed a liking for the simpler patterns, the two variables, liking and "interestingness," do not appear to be closely related, and what relationship there is appears to be inverse.

Summary of Tartan Studies. This set of materials was selected because it offered a physical dimension, number of squares, with a degree of face validity as a complexity dimension. The physical scale and a simple psychological rating scale showed good agreement.

The relation of complexity and liking was a simple monotonic one, with subjects expressing the greater liking for the simpler patterns. Ratings of "interestingness" and ratings of liking were essentially unrelated.

Comparison of a simple scaling of liking and results from a more complex

Shepard-Kruskal scaling technique yielded no advantage of the more complex technique, either in terms of the establishment of more than one dimension of liking, or in terms of individual difference analysis.

State Set Designs§

The design of stage settings is subject to classification with respect to style, and the various styles differ in complexity as one of the descriptive dimensions. In conjunction with a doctoral dissertation on differences in audience reaction to styles of stage setting, a group of 30 photographs of drawings of stage sets became available.

This group of 30 photographs was subjected to two kinds of preliminary appraisal. They were submitted to a panel of scholars in drama for quantitative evaluation of the extent to which each represented any of several styles. They were also rated by a small group of subjects for complexity and preference, using a simple rating procedure. On the basis of these two preliminary procedures, a set of 12 drawings was selected for use in the dissertation. The criterion of choice was primarily that the panel of scholars be in agreement on the style designations.

The settings selected represented three styles, romantic, classical or formal, and baroque. The romantic settings were: one by Chaperon for Faust, one by Adolph Appia for Little Eyolf, one by Karl Fichot for Parsifal, and one by P. L. Ciceri for Ali Baba. The formal or classical settings were: one from Karl Czeschka for King Lear, one from Norman Bel Geddes for Hamlet, one from T. C. Pillartz for Oedipus, and one from Adolph Appia for Orpheus. The baroque settings included one from Fabrizio Galliari, one from Ferdinando Bibiena, and two from Carlo Bibiena. The plays for which they were designed were not designated in the source.

The 12 stage set drawings were then rated four different times by a group of subjects consisting of nine undergraduate and seven graduate students. They were rated for complexity and preference on a simple 7-point scale and rated for both variables, again using the Shepard-Kruskal technique.

The results of the simple rating are shown in FIGURE 7. The three styles are distinguished in terms of complexity almost without overlap. The four baroque settings are rated as much more complex than the others. The four classical-formal settings are rated on the simple end of the scale. The romantic are in the middle except for one setting that is classed with the formal in terms of complexity.

These subjects express a preference for the baroque settings. The classical-formal are least preferred, but the styles are not differentiated in terms of preference to nearly the extent they are in terms of complexity. Thus, the realtionship between complexity and preference is a monotonically increasing preference for settings of increasing complexity. It might be noted that this is the reverse of the relationship between complexity and preference noted in the studies of tartan patterns.

The Shepard-Kruskal ratings were extensively analyzed, using up to six dimensions in both the analyses of individual data and in the analysis of the group data. Again, the efforts to rationalize the individual data proved utterly fruitless. The analysis of group data was equally frustrating. When the Shepard-

§ This study was done in conjunction with a doctoral dissertation project of Warren Pickett in the Department of Speech and Drama at the University of Michigan. The dissertation, tentatively titled An Experiment in Audience Response to Set Design Style, is to be completed in the Fall term, 1969.

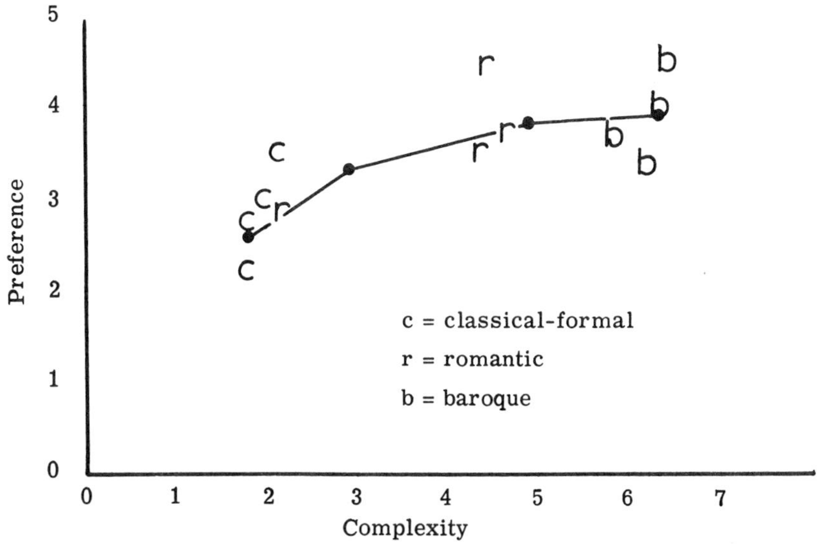

FIGURE 7. Complexity and preference in stage set designs (7-point scales).

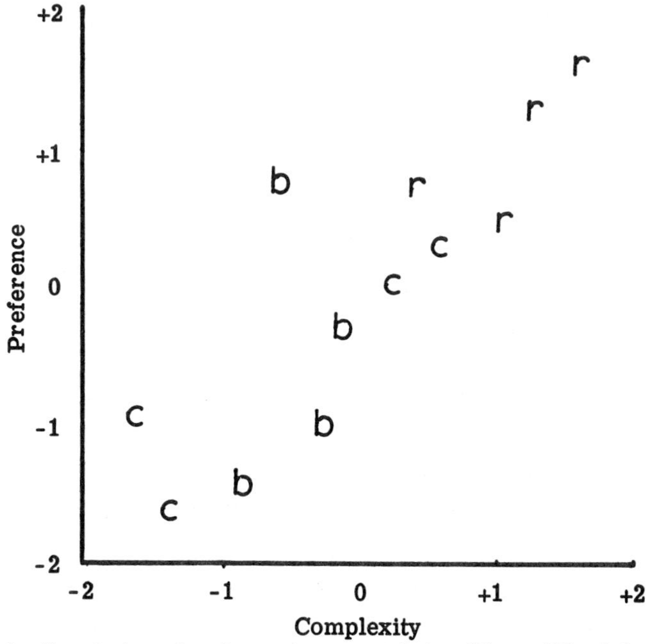

FIGURE 8. Complexity and preference in stage set designs (Shepard-Kruskal scales).

Kruskal analyses of complexity were compared with the results of the 7-point scale, the only systematic relationship that emerged was a U-shaped relationship with one of the Shepard-Kruskal dimensions. Sets rated both high and low in complexity on the 7-point scale were at one end of the Shepard-Kruskal dimension, and those in the middle were on the other end.

With six dimensions of complexity and six of preference available, 30 possible pairs can be matched. FIGURE 8 is a plot of the one pairing that showed a systematic relationship. This plot is so linear that one would think that the two dimensions were measurements of the same variable. The other possibility is that this relationship is a chance one drawn from a set of 30.

The methodological conclusion drawn from these efforts is that the simple rating scale functions as well or better than the more complex multidimensional one, since the latter added no information concerning either variable or the relation between the two.

Complexity, Preference, and Experience with Graphics¶

Theories that relate preference to stimulus complexity generally agree in predicting that a subject will prefer a stimulus of moderate complexity rather than an extremely simple or an extremely complex stimulus. The theory stated earlier predicts that with increased experience with a class of stimuli, the preferred stimulus should tend to be chosen from a point closer to the more complex end of the scale.

This study is an attempt to verify the existence of an optimal complexity level in the middle range of a scale of complexity and to determine if the optimal point is higher for subjects with more experience with the range of stimuli. The basic design was to choose a set of graphics that are highly representational in character and that were produced by well-known artists. These were then rated for complexity and preference by a group of law students who were naive with respect to graphic prints, a group of art history students, and a group of graduate students in art. The latter two groups could be expected to recognize many, if not all, of the graphics and to be able to identify the artist in each case.

The first step in the process was to choose 30 prints of graphic art by seven recognized artists. All of the prints were black and white, were the same size (4.5″ × 5″) mounted on slightly larger white cardboards and covered with clear acetate for protection.

In the first phase of the study, this set of 30 prints was given to 40 subjects, individually. The group of subjects was equally divided between students in law school and students in either art or art history. They were asked to look through the entire set and then to assign a whole number rating of complexity from 1 to 7.

Mean ratings for the 30 prints were then used as a basis for choosing a set of 15 prints for the second phase of the study. Five prints each were chosen from the high, mid-, and low portions of the range of ratings, with the additional prescription that the standard deviations of the ratings should be minimal.

In the second phase of the study, 60 subjects forming three groups of 20 subjects each were used. A "naive" group consisted of 20 law students with little experience with graphic materials of the kind used in the study. Few of these subjects were able to recognize any of the prints or identify any of the artists. An "art" group was composed of 20 senior or graduate students in art. An "art history" group was composed of 20 graduate students majoring in art history.

¶ This study was planned and executed by Kathleen Sinclair and submitted as an Honors Thesis entitled Optimal Complexity and Aesthetic Preference, University of Michigan, 1967.

That the "art" and "art history" groups had had considerably more experience with the stimulus materials is demonstrated by the fact that all of the members of both groups recognized all of the artists and most of the prints used in the study. The list of prints ordered from most to least complex in terms of the mean complexity score obtained in the first phase of the study is contained in TABLE 2.

The complexity ratings are reasonably stable. The correlation (rho) between

TABLE 2

LIST OF GRAPHIC PRINTS*

Mean Complexity Rating	Artist and Title of Print
6.4	Durer, "The Men's Bath"
6.2	Durer, "The Sea-Monster," 1500
5.9	Breughel, "The Donkey at School," 1556
5.6	Durer, "Les Trois Graces," 1491
4.3	Durer, "Portrait of the Artist's Mother," 1514
4.0	Chagall, "David Gives Vent to his Grief," 1931
3.95	Toulouse-Lautrec, "La Goulue au Moulin Rouge," 1891
3.9	Goya, "Self Destruction," 1800
3.7	Toulouse-Lautrec, "La Goulue avec une Tanseur," 1891
3.6	Picasso, "The Ball," 1904
2.7	Matisse, "Portrait of Prof. T. Whitmore," 1937
2.6	Chagall, "The Musician," 1919
2.4	Chagall, "My Mother," 1919
1.5	Matisse, "The Princess N"
1.4	Matisse, "Henri de Montherlant," 1937

* The prints that were rated by subjects for complexity and preference in the second phase of the study are arranged in order of the mean complexity values obtained in the first phase.

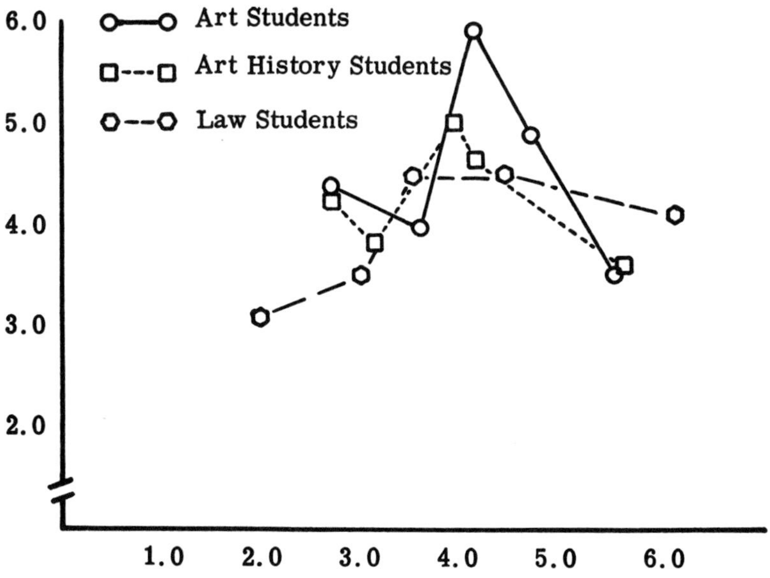

FIGURE 9. Optimal complexity and experience.

the ratings in two phases is .94. The correlations among the complexity ratings given by the three groups are .93, .94, and .94.

FIGURE 9 was achieved by ordering the 15 complexity values and grouping them in sets of three. Means were obtained for each set of three, and the mean preference value for each set was then obtained. The curves in FIGURE 9 are obviously different, and the differences are statistically significant. The curve for the naive subjects is relative flat and they tend to use most of the range of complexity. However, the flatness of the curve indicates that they do not show very consistent preferences except that there is a general preference for the more complex end of the scale. The curves for the more sophisticated subjects are constricted in range on the complexity scale. They tend to see the graphics in a context that makes them more nearly alike in complexity. Both curves show major preference for the middle range of complexity values, an optimum in the middle of the range.

The location of the optimum as a function of the amount of experience is in the direction predicted by the theory. The art history students have considerably less experience with graphics than do the graduate students in art. The arts students show an optimum that is to the right of that for the art history students. However, this apparent difference is not sufficiently great to accept as evidence. A clear demonstration of the movement of the optimum up the complexity scale with increased experience is yet to be demonstrated unequivocally with these materials.

Modern Art. Our most extensive work on measurement techniques and methodology was devoted to the development of a set of materials representing modern abstract art. A large set of stimulus materials was prepared, and from this set, 42 abstract paintings were selected. These were all in color and were abstract in the sense of being nonrepresentational and generally devoid of symbolic material. TABLE 3 contains a list of the paintings used in the preliminary study. The objective was to develop a standardized set of stimulus materials that would then be available for use in studies of complexity and preference, especially studies involving extensive exposure and possible changes in preference with exposure.

The tasks given to subjects involved making four ratings of the paintings. They were to rate complexity and preference on seven-point scales. Then they were to perform the Shepard-Kruskal scaling task, rating differences in complexity or preference between pairs on a scale of 1 to 10. With 42 stimulus items, the task of rating all possible pairs twice, once for complexity and once for preference, proved to be almost beyond the patience of willing subjects. They complained about the difficulty of the task and the growing unpleasantness. Fifteen subjects agreed to perform the scaling task, and only seven completed the entire sequence of judgments. Each of these seven subjects was then interviewed at length concerning the bases of choices. This interview provided a lengthy protocol against which to compare the scales derived.

The abstract paintings are rich in complexity. They vary in color, technique, degree of homogeneity of line and shape, number of transitions from one color or brightness to another, suggestiveness of meaningful material, and so on. It was felt that ratings of complexity and preference with such materials might well be multidimensional. If they did prove to be multidimensional, the Shepard-Kruskal analysis should reveal dimensions that could be matched against the verbal protocol for each subject.

The general procedure in pursuing this objective was to obtain Shepard-Kruskal analyses from the computer in a number of degrees of detail. Thus, for each subject, the computer generated ten sets of solutions for one dimension through ten

TABLE 3

MODERN ABSTRACT PAINTINGS

Set Number	7-point Complexity Rating	Painter	Painting	Year
1	5.6	Jackson Pollack	#1	1949
	4.5	Jo Schreiter	Execution of the hope	1957
	4.1	Singier	Les Amoureux et la Plage	1954
G	3.2	Sugai'	Yamato	1956
	3.5	Tobey	Tatouage	1958
2	6.1	Singier	L'Eté	1945
3	3.4	Hofmann	Pompei	1959
4	2.4	Sugai'	Yayoi	1958
5	5.8	Willi Baumeister	Animated landscape	1946
	2.5	Stamos	Avignon II	1958
6	1.4	Piet Mondriaan	Composition	1927
	4.5	Max Ackermann	Jubilation	1954
F	3.4	Piet Mondriaan	Composition	1913
7	5.5	Corneille	Tropical splendour	1958
8	5.3	Wassily Kandinsky	Pink Composition	
9	2.3	Soulages	Peinture	1957
	4.9	Corneille	Landscape of America	1958
	2.4	Dubuffet	Table	1957
E	4.7	Vieira Da Silva	Red Interior	1951
10	5.5	Marca-Relli	Summer noon	1956
	4.4	Bram Van Velde	Composition Collection Marie Cuttoli	1957
	4.9	Bram Van Velde	Composition	1957
	4.0	Lyonel Feininger	Month of R. Rega III	
11	6.4	Goodnough	Summer	1959–60
12	2.1	Stamos	Persian Bride	1958
13	4.3	Le Moal	Ocean	1959
D	3.3	Singier	Soleil et sable	1956
	3.3	Sugai'	Oni	1958
14	5.1	Prassinos	Le Clown	1960
15	1.5	Mark Rothko	Number 10	1950
C	4.5	Schneider	Peinture 65 B	1954
B	5.8	Dubuffet	Garden Bleche Grignotte	1956
16	3.8	Poliakoff	Oil	1953
17	2.8	Sugai'	Sugata	1958
18	3.5	Schneider	Peinture 95 B	1955
19	4.4	Tobey	Intersection	1954
	4.1	Tobey	Pacific Circle	1956
	3.5	Soulages	Peinture	1958
20	3.0	Pierre Soulages	Composition	
	4.3	Tobey	Summer	1957
21	3.9	Goetz	Peinture	1954
A	2.8	Tobey	Yellow Harvest	1956

dimensions, i.e., 55 dimensions for complexity and 55 for preference for each of 7 subjects.

Analyses of the data for an individual subject tended to take the following form. The one-dimensional solutions and the two dimensions of the two-dimensional solutions for complexity and preference were plotted for every individual, and many pairings of higher level were plotted. The resulting plots varied in the extent of apparent relations, but examination of a large number of such plots revealed nothing that was meaningfully different from the later analysis of the group data. The second step was to use the Shepard-Kruskal dimensions in pairs to arrange the paintings in two-dimensional arrays. A room wall was utilized for this purpose. A vertical scale was fastened to the wall from floor to ceiling, and a horizontal scale was fastened to the wall from left to right. Then, for example, the two dimensional Shepard-Kruskal solution for an individual subject would be used to place each of the 42 paintings on the wall in accordance with its assigned values from the analysis. If the scales were complexity scales, then the array would be examined to see whether there was any way of making sense of the dimensions in terms of complexity. If the array represented preference, then they

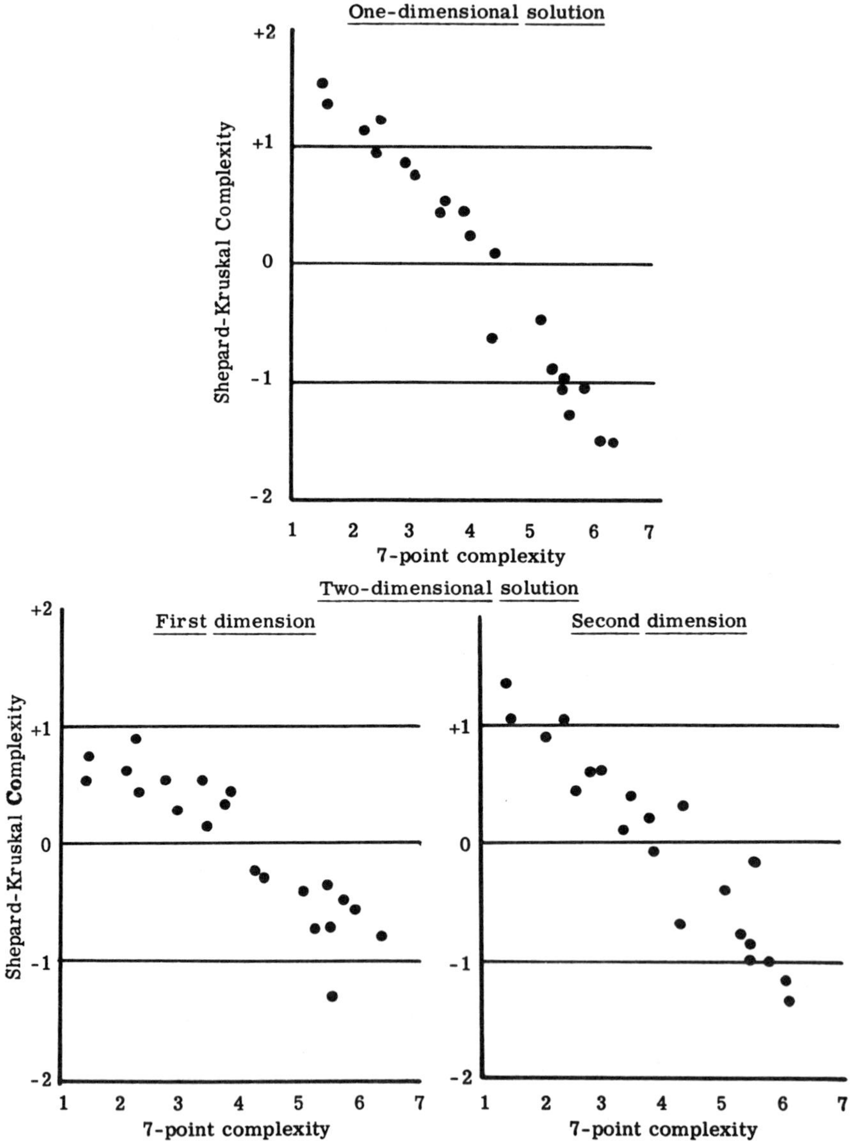

FIGURE 10. Comparison of 7-point and Shepard-Kruskal scales of complexity.

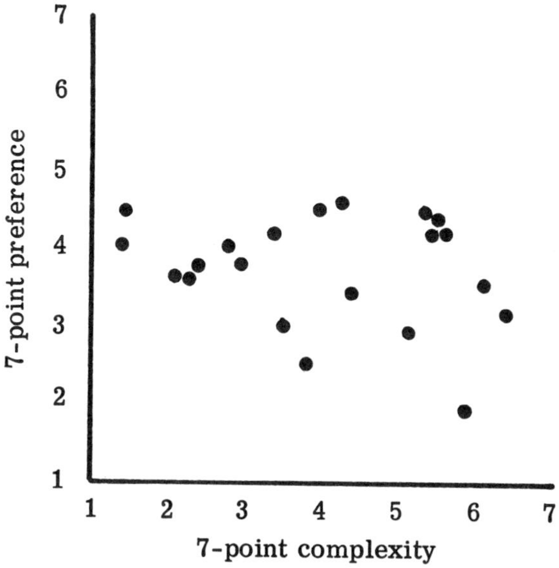

FIGURE 11. Complexity versus preference for modern paintings (7-point scale data).

were examined to ascertain whether the basis of preference along each of the dimensions could be determined. These examinations were aided by the protocols taken from the subjects in an effort to determine why a given painting should occupy that particular position in the array. Several experimenters spent a great many hours at this task. Many arrays were examined by as many as seven or eight people. Many arrays were photographed in color and examined later in an effort to establish meaningfulness. Although it was not done systematically, a number of arrays was examined by the subjects who had provided the original data. The net outcome was the conclusion that multidimensional analyses of these data did not yield more than one dimension of either complexity or preference in the data of individual subjects.

For a variety of reasons, it was decided that working with 42 stimuli was unnecessarily cumbersome. The mean 7-point complexity values for the 15 subjects was then used to reduce the set of 42 paintings to a set of 21 experimental paintings and a practice set of six. TABLE 3 contains the mean complexity values. It also contains the code number assigned to the 21 paintings of the experimental set, and the letters A through G for the practice set that could be used in instructing future subjects.

This small set was then rated by 15 subjects, on both 7-point and Shepard-Kruskal scales in an effort to determine the extent of agreement of the two scaling techniques and whether any advantage accrued from the use of the more complicated Shepard-Kruskal procedure.

FIGURE 10 shows a comparison of the 7-point ratings of complexity compared to the one-dimensional and both dimensions of the two-dimensional Shepard-Kruskal solutions. In all three cases there is good agreement in these grouped data. If a stimulus is rated complex on one scale, it is likely to be rated as complex by use of the other method. The two dimensions of the two-dimensional

Shepard-Kruskal solution both show good agreement, suggesting that they are highly correlated dimensions within the Shepard-Kruskal analysis.

FIGURE 11 is a plot of the 7-point complexity and preference values. Almost no trend is apparent in the data beyond a minor tendency for mean preference for some of the more complex stimuli to be somewhat low. FIGURE 12 shows a comparison of the Shepard-Kruskal one dimensional solutions for complexity and preference. Again, no reliable trend is apparent.

FIGURE 13 contains the plots of 7-point complexity ratings and three Shepard-Kruskal dimensions of preference. None shows relationships.

Two conclusions seem justified on the basis of these studies. The first is that it seems probably that when one asks a subject to rate a set of abstract paintings for complexity or preference, the subject does just that. It is a simple pair of dimensions from the standpoint of the subject and it is thus not composed of contributing sets of underlying dimensions. The second conclusion is that in these data, no systematic relationship between complexity and preference could be demonstrated.

A possible explanation for the lack of relationship between complexity and preference in these data might lie in the experience factor. The theory of complexity predicts that there will be changes in complexity and preference with experience. It could be that such changes were occurring rapidly enough that the mean judgments represented valid judgments from different points in time that were not coordinate because of the order or presentation and the amount of experience provided in the experimental situation.

Based on this possibility, an effort was made to introduce a simple control of experience within the setting and collect a new set of data with a larger number

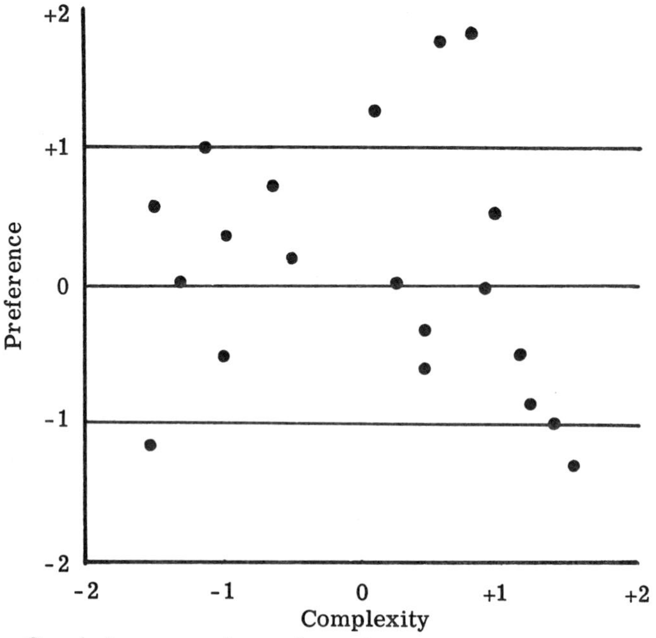

FIGURE 12. Complexity versus preference for modern paintings (Shepard-Kruskal scale data).

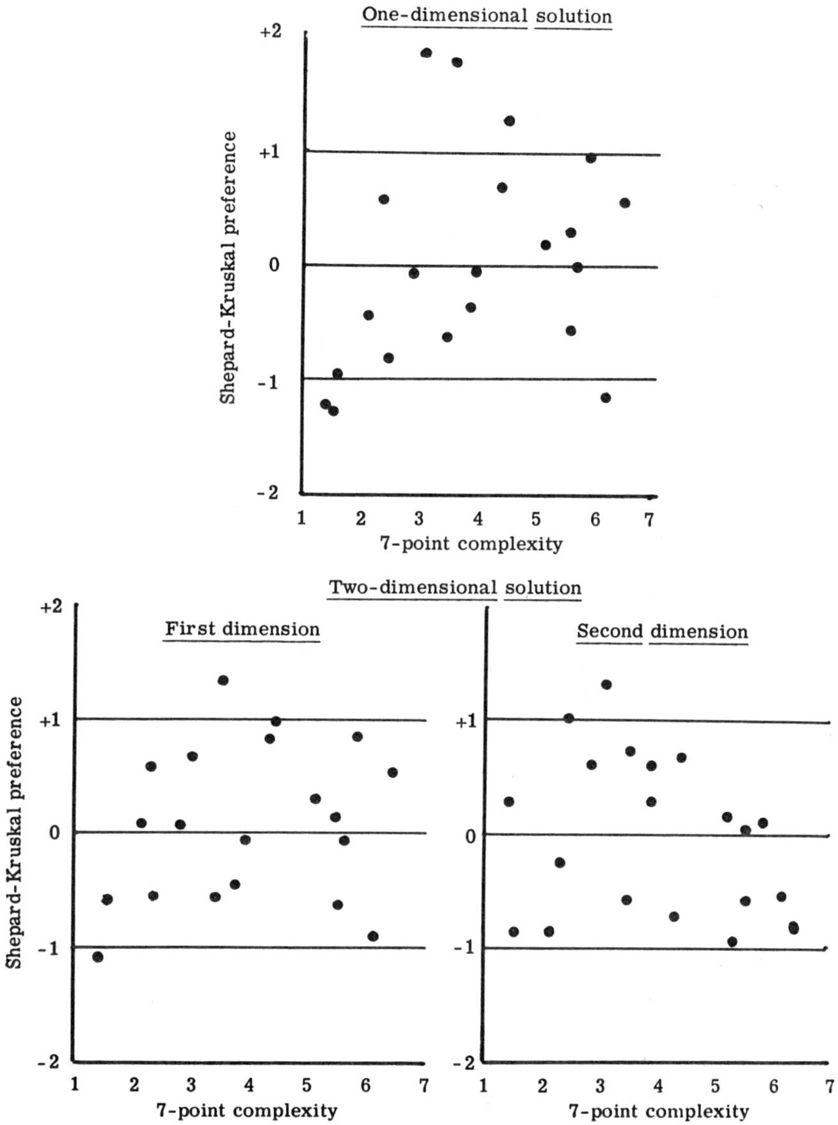

FIGURE 13. Complexity versus preference for modern paintings (7-point scales of complexity versus Shepard-Kruskal preference solutions).

of subjects. The simple 7-point scaling procedure was used. The demonstration set of six paintings was used to explain the procedure. The 40 subjects were then asked to rate each of the 21 pictures for complexity and preference.

The major results in terms of complexity and preference is plotted in FIGURE 14. There is a definite relation between the two, with preference being expressed for the more complex of the paintings.

Summary of Results from Human Studies of Complexity and Preference

The major effort in this area was to develop several sets of visual stimulus materials for use in future research. The research has produced four sets, each of which yields reliable ratings of complexity and preference.

The methodological conclusions are simple and somewhat disappointing. Multidimensional analysis of ratings of complexity and preference does not seem fruitful. The simplest rating tasks, in which the subject is asked to assign an absolute rating from 1 to 7, from 1 to 10, or from 1 to 100, seem to yield results that are as functional for future research as the more complex scaling techniques. The Shepard-Kruskal technique imposes a very difficult task on the subject and requires that the subject be exposed to the stimuli a number of times and for considerable periods. It seems likely that the complexity value and preference for the stimuli are undergoing extensive change during the process of rating.

The search for an optimum preference value along the complexity dimension yielded rather varied results. The "best'" result with each of the four sets of stimulus materials is plotted in FIGURE 15. Subjects express maximum preference for the simplest of the tartan patterns. They show a maximum preference for black and white graphics in the middle range of complexity. Maximum preference is expressed for the most complex of the stage settings and the abstract paintings.

The effect of experience on complexity and preference was explored systematically in only one study. In that one, the more experienced art students used a more restricted range of complexity ratings and a wider range of preference ratings than did the more naive subjects. Optimal preference for middle values of complexity was evident in this study, but a significant increase in the complexity of optimal preference with experience was not demonstrated.

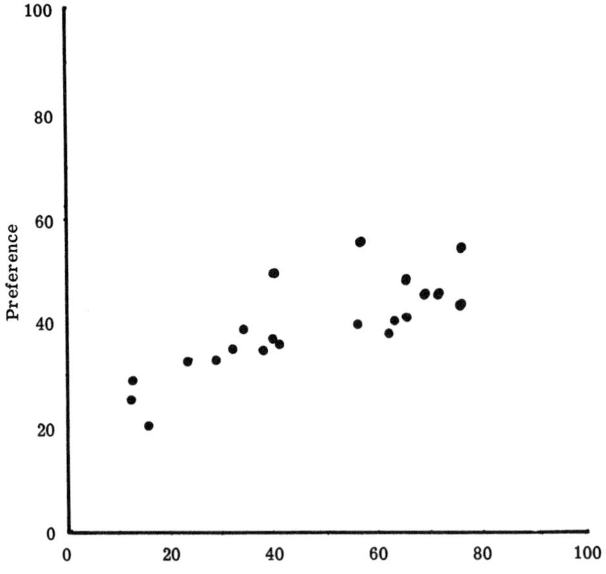

FIGURE 14. Complexity versus preference for modern paintings.

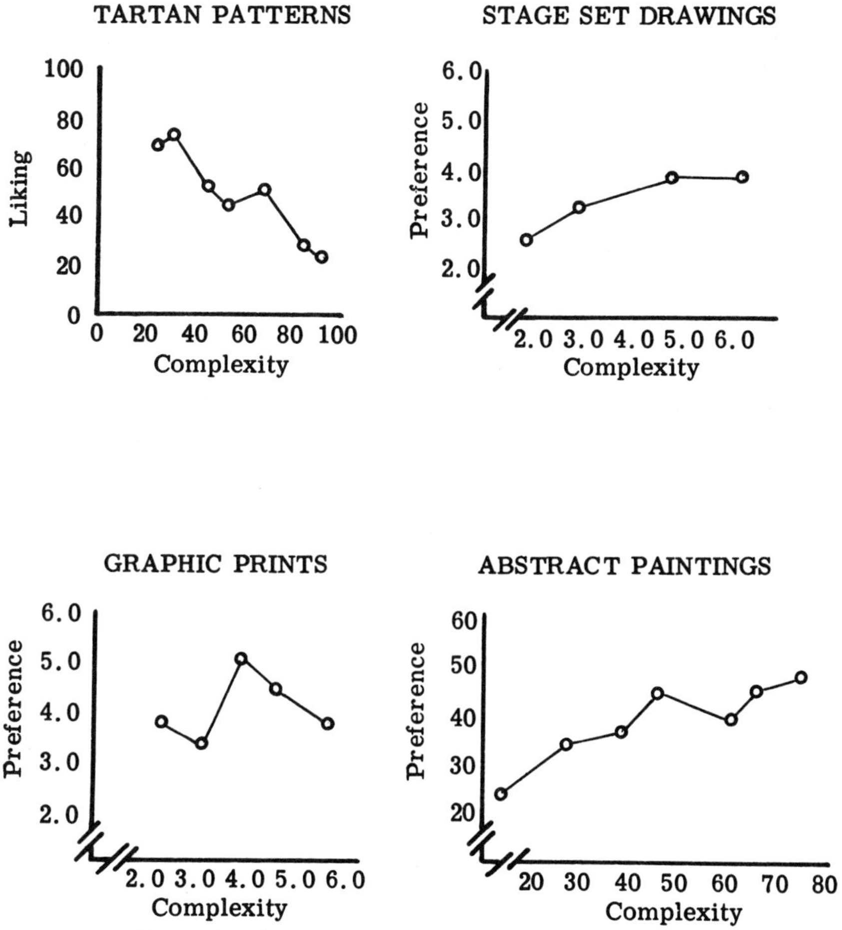

FIGURE 15. Summary of complexity and preference relations.

STIMULUS COMPLEXITY AND PREFERENCE IN ANIMALS

It is easy to ask a human subject how complex he thinks a given stimulus is and then to ask him to rate his preference for it. It is more difficult to have an animal try to distinguish between the two questions. If one presents an array of stimuli to an animal and if the animal approaches one element of that array, it is reasonable to assume that he prefers that stimulus to the others. If the array is composed of stimuli that have a dimension of complexity that is obvious to the experimenter, then one can infer that the animal has expressed a preference for the chosen stimulus on the basis of its relative complexity. However, the inference is not a strong one. If, in the pattern of successive choices, the animal behaves in a manner that is orderly along this complexity dimension, the inference that it is the complexity of the stimulus to which he is responding seems strengthened.

The lack of independence of the judgments of complexity and preference is the major disadvantage of working with animals on this problem. The advantage lies in the assumed relative simplicity of the animal and the degree of control that the experimenter can exercise. Animal research on complexity and preference was undertaken in the light of the obvious advantages and disadvantages.

Two-dimensional versus three-dimensional complexity in the rat. The first study of this series[8] was an effort to explore the question whether repeated experience with two sets of stimuli (two dimensional and three-dimensional) would produce a progressively changing preference toward more complex stimuli. One stimulus set consisted of simple wall patterns composed of (1) a uniform grey, (2) a set of horizontal stripes, (3) a set of vertical stripes, and (4) a checkered pattern. The three-dimensional patterns consisted of (1) an empty compartment, (2) a compartment with one baffle, (3) a compartment with two baffles, and (4) a compartment with a complex set of baffles greater than two. It was assumed that these two sets of stimuli represented two dimensions of complexity, both of which were anchored on the empty grey compartment.

A group of 16 animals was run in each maze. They were run individually and left in the maze for a period of 30 minutes on each of five successive days. The sequence of choices and time spent in each compartment were recorded.

The compartment in which an animal spends more time than any other can be designated as his preferred compartment for that day. TABLE 4 is a tabulation of preferred compartment for each day for each group. The stimuli are ordered in the Table in the *a priori* order of complexity with respect to which they were designed.||

TABLE 4

PREFERRED COMPARTMENTS BY DAYS

		Wall Patterns		
Days	Grey	Horizontal Stripes	Vertical Stripes	Checks
1	16	0	0	0
2	16	0	0	0
3	14	1	1	0
4	13	2	1	0
5	7.5	1	3.5	4
		Baffle Patterns		
Days	Grey	One Baffle	Two Baffles	Three-plus baffles
1	0	6.5	4.5	5
2	1	2	0	13
3	0	0	1	15
4	0	1	0	15
5	0	1	0.5	14.5

In the wall pattern maze, the simplest compartment with grey walls is preferred by every animal for the first two days. On subsequent days, increasing number of animals express preference for increasingly complex wall patterns. In the baffle maze, preference is expressed about equally for the three more complex patterns on the first day. By the second day the animals are almost universally expressing a preference for the most complex of the quadrants.

Some of the problems of interpretation of these results may be seen more clearly if the data are plotted on a hypothetical scale of stimulus complexity. This has been done in FIGURE 16. Each number represents the mean preference for the

|| The analyses presented here differ slightly from those presented in reference 8.

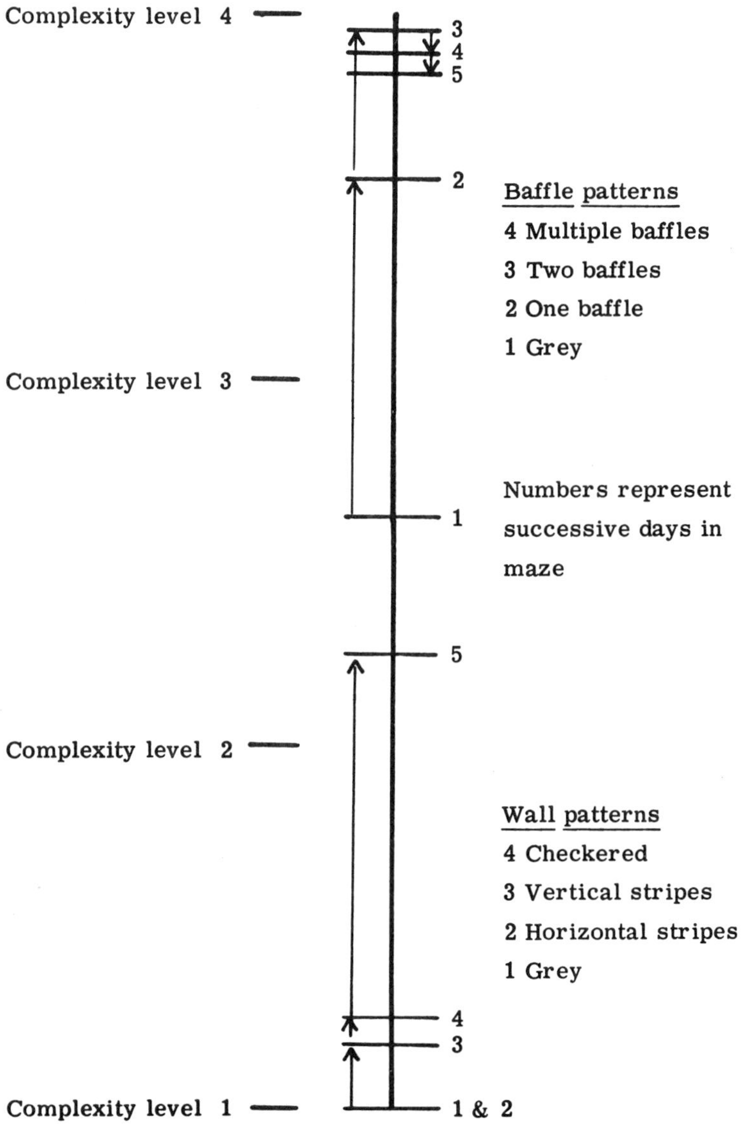

FIGURE 16. Stimulus complexity scale.

day (number of animals × the arbitrary complexity value/N). The animals exposed to the wall patterns show a predominant preference for the grey compartment on the first two days, then move to a slight preference for more complex patterns on the third and fourth days, and make a significant shift upward only on the fifth day. The animals with the baffle patterns show a preference midway on the scale on the first day, and move very close to the top by the second.

The scale in FIGURE 16 is dependent on the arbitrary assignment of complexity scale values of "1" for the grey compartment in each case, a value of "2" for the next most complex, and a value of "3" and the "4" for the next two. These values assume equal metric values for the horizontal stripes and for the one baffle, equal value for vertical stripes and two baffles, and equal weights for the checkered pattern and the multiple baffles. Without an appeal to the theory there is no simple way to determine which set of stimuli, the two-dimensional or the three-dimensional, is the more complex.

If we take the theory seriously, then we could reason in the following fashion. Since the animals took several days to venture at all into the more complex two-dimensional patterns in contrast to the immediate approach to the baffle patterns, then the wall patterns are probably the more complex and should be assigned complexity values greater than those assigned the baffle patterns. However, there is no simple way to determine what scale values to assign to the stimuli.

An alternative is to combine into one maze representatives of the two types of stimuli. To do this, the same maze compartments were redesigned with the following stimulus patterns.**

1. Grey walls, no baffles
2. Grey walls, one baffle
3. Horizontal stripe walls, no baffles
4. Vertical stripe walls, three baffles

The first of these, the grey walls without baffles, seemed to be an obvious choice for the simplest stimulus pattern we could devise. The fourth, the vertical striped pattern with the three baffles was a combination of the two most complex of the two previous sets of stimuli. The other two seemed to be middle values. If one had to guess, on the basis of previous results, one would guess that the one baffle pattern would be the simpler of the two.

Only three rats were used in the study, but each of the three was exposed to the stimuli for continuous sessions of 100 minutes each on six consecutive days. It was hoped that the much longer exposure times would be adequate to permit significant changes in preference.

In order to analyze the data, each session was arbitrarily divided into ten periods of ten minutes each. For each such time block, the quadrant in which the animal spent the majority of his time was designated as the preferred compartment.

TABLE 5 is a tabulation of the number of blocks out of 30 (ten each for three animals) in which each quadrant was preferred, on each of the six days. The data are generally orderly, in spite of the small number of animals. The initial preference is clearly for the simplest of the quadrants, and the final preference clearly for the most complex. The guess that the baffle pattern would be less complex than the horizontal stripes seems supported by the fact that the preference for the horizontal stripes is expressed later in the time sequence.

The data can be analyzed within days as well. This has been done in TABLE 6. Again, the data seem orderly despite the handicap of the small number of animals and the fact that the preference is changing markedly from day to day, as shown in TABLE 5. Looking down the columns, the preference for the one baffle quadrant declines in the 100-minute period, while the preference for the two more complex patterns increases slightly. Looking across the rows, the theory would state that the pattern one would not expect would be one that declined and then in-

** This study was done by Bruce E. Walker and is unpublished. Its title might be Scaling of Two-Dimensional and Three-Dimensional Stimulus Complexity in the Rat.

TABLE 5

PREFERRED STIMULI BY DAYS

Day	Grey	1 Baffle	Horizontal Stripes	Vertical Stripes and 3 Baffles
1	20	9	0	1
2	6	17	7	0
3	1	15	14	0
4	2	12	12	4
5	2	13	5	10
6	0	8	7	15

TABLE 6

PREFERRED STIMULI BY SUCCESSIVE TEN-MINUTE PERIODS

Minutes	Grey	1 Baffle	Horizontal Stripes	Vertical Stripes and 3 Baffles
1– 10	2	14	0	2
11– 20	1	11	4	2
21– 30	4	9	3	2
31– 40	3	9	4	2
41– 50	5	6	5	2
51- 60	4	6	6	2
61- 70	2	6	7	3
71– 80	4	3	6	5
81– 90	3	5	5	5
91–100	3	5	5	5

creased. In only two of the 30 instances is the expectation not met. Thus there is a general tendency for the animals to move from less complex to more complex stimuli during the day.

Analysis of Sequences of Choice. The theory relating complexity and preference indicates that the expressed preference should be for progressively more complex stimuli. In the simplest form of the theory, there should be no regressions. That is, if an animal first prefers the grey compartment and then progresses to a preference for the compartment with one baffle, he should not again express a preference for the plain grey compartment. The prediction does not contain a statement concerning variability or error. It simply states that if we number the quadrants from 1 through 4, the preference sequence should be 1, 2, 3, 4, and no sequence such as 1, 2, 3, 2, 3, 4 should be observed. Rigid adherence to the complexity sequence seems too much to expect, yet the theory makes no prediction related to the variability in the sequence.

Analysis of sequences has an inherent problem. One way of analyzing the data would be to list a sequence of choices, in this case compartment entries, and then analyze the sequence for sequential dependencies. However, such a sequence of choices would not take the amount of time spent in each compartment into account. An alternative analysis would simply be the total amount of time spent in each compartment. This analysis yields no information on sequences of choices. A compromise analysis is in terms of arbitrary time blocks. In this case, one can use the ten-minute time blocks that were used in the previous analysis. For each time block, the quadrant in which the animal spent the most time can be designated as the preferred stimulus for that time block. Such an analysis loses data on brief visits and differs slightly from analyses in terms of total time spent in each quadrant. However, it does have the advantage of representing the sequence of choices made and the time spent in each compartment and, therefore, in the presence of each stimulus.

In this study, if one takes the sequences of designations of preferred stimuli for each animal over the six days, the sequences consist of 60 successive designations of preferred stimulus for each animal. Each sequence can then be analyzed by tabulating the frequency with which each designation of preference is followed by each other designation. The frequencies can then be converted to first-order transitional probabilities. This has been done for each animal in TABLE 7. It has been done for all three animals but for Days 1 and 2, Days 3 and 4, and Days 5 and 6 in pairs in TABLE 8. TABLE 8 also contains the summary table of transitional probabilities for all six days for all three animals.

The major individual differences in TABLE 7 are that Animal X rarely entered the most complex quadrant with the vertical stripes and the multiple baffles. Animal Y, on the other hand, visited the horizontal striped compartment rather infrequently. If the complexity ordering in the Table is correct, this animal jumped directly from the one-baffle pattern to the most complex. There appears to be no simple way to unfold a scale based on nothing but sequences to order the stimuli for individual animals, but it could be that for Animal Y, the complexity order of the one-baffle and the horizontal stripes is reversed from the order in the Table.

The analysis of transitional probabilities by days in TABLE 8 shows a clear progression given the *a priori* ordering of the stimulus patterns. The action is relatively confined to the two simpler stimuli on the first two days. It moves to the second and third stimuli on the next two days, and progresses to include the most complex stimulus on the final two days.

While complexity theory does not predict the amount of variability in choice

TABLE 7

TRANSITIONAL PROBABILITIES OF STIMULUS PREFERENCE BY ANIMAL

		TO: Grey	One Baffle	Horizontal Stripes	Stripes & Baffles
Animal X					
FROM	Grey	.08	.07	.00	.00
	One Baffle	.05	.17	.05	.00
	Horizontal St.	.00	.05	.44	.03
	Stripes & Baffles	.02	.00	.02	.00
Animal Y					
FROM	Grey	.08	.02	.00	.00
	One Baffle	.02	.41	.03	.07
	Horizontal St.	.00	.03	.05	.00
	Stripes & Baffles	.02	.03	.00	.24
Animal Z					
FROM	Grey	.15	.08	.02	.00
	One Baffle	.07	.29	.03	.03
	Horizontal St.	.03	.02	.12	.00
	Stripes & Baffles	.00	.02	.00	.14

TABLE 8

CHANGING PREFERENCES FOR STIMULUS COMPLEXITIES OVER TIME IN TERMS OF TRANSITIONAL PROBABILITIES

		Grey	One Baffle	Horizontal Stripes	Stripes & Baffles
		Days 1 and 2 TO			
FROM	Grey	.34	.11	.00	.00
	One Baffle	.12	.27	.04	.02
	Horizontal St.	.00	.02	.09	.00
	Stripes & Baffles	.02	.00	.00	.00
		Days 3 and 4 TO			
FROM	Grey	.00	.04	.02	.00
	One Baffle	.02	.37	.05	.02
	Horizontal St.	.04	.02	.37	.02
	Stripes & Baffles	.00	.00	.02	.04
		Days 4 and 5 TO			
FROM	Grey	.00	.04	.02	.00
	One Baffle	.02	.23	.02	.09
	Horizontal St.	.00	.02	.18	.00
	Stripes & Baffles	.02	.05	.00	.34
		Days 1 through 6 TO			
FROM	Grey	.11	.06	.01	.00
	One Baffle	.05	.29	.04	.03
	Horizontal St.	.01	.03	.20	.01
	Stripes & Baffles	.01	.02	.01	.12

sequence one might expect, it does make some predictions concerning a table such as that on the bottom of TABLE 8. If the progression of preferences was ordered absolutely, then all of the probabilities of the table would be along the diagonal except for three transitions, from 1 to 2, from 2 to 3, and from 3 to 4, and there should be no reversals, e.g. from 3 to 2. It is apparent that the preference sequences are not ordered absolutely.

A weaker prediction would be that the transitional probabilities would depart from a chance distribution. It is obvious, without test, that this prediction is fulfilled. The theory also makes a prediction concerning the character of the dependency. If the animals are responding to the stimuli and are reacting to them as they have been ordered on an *a priori* basis, then the interaction between adjacent stimuli should be greater than more remote stimuli. The sum of the probabilities in the diagonals adjacent to the main diagonal is .20. The sum of the more remote interactions (the three in the lower left and the three in the upper right) is .08. This result would tend to confirm that the animals were indeed responding to the complexity scale and that they were responding to it as it is ordered in the Tables.

Generalized Complexity Satiation.§§ Complexity theory predicts that with continued exposure to a stimulus dimension, the organism should show preference for

§§ This study was carried out by Bruce E. Walker and is unpublished. It might be titled Effect of Prior Exposure to One Stimulus on Preference for Other Stimuli on the Same Dimension.

stimuli of increasing complexity, and this prediction has been repeatedly verified in the previous studies. If there is generalization of the effects of exposure to one stimulus on a dimension, it should have an influence on the relative preference for stimuli on the same dimension to which the organism has not been exposed.

To test this proposition, a study was designed in the following pattern. Five stimuli were constructed that should represent a dimension of stimulus complexity to the rat. The five patterns were all vertical stripe patterns of black and white and they varied in width. The widths were:

Most complex	3/16-inch stripes
	3/8-inch stripes
Middle complexity	3/4-inch stripes
	1 & 1/2-inch stripes
Least complex	3-inch stripes

The basic plan was to vary the amount of prior exposure of groups of animals to the middle stimulus and then to observe the effect of the different durations of exposure on the preferences of the animals when given choices among the other four.

It was felt that the total amount of exposure in the maze should be held constant, in this case at one hour, but that the duration of exposure to the 3/4-inch stripe pattern should be varied. To do this, the four-compartment maze was employed, and all three groups were initially placed in the maze with the walls a uniform grey. A short exposure group was created by leaving the animals in the grey condition for 50 minutes, removing them while the stripe pattern was installed, and then putting them back for ten minutes to complete the hour of exposure. A middle exposure group was created by exposing them to the grey for

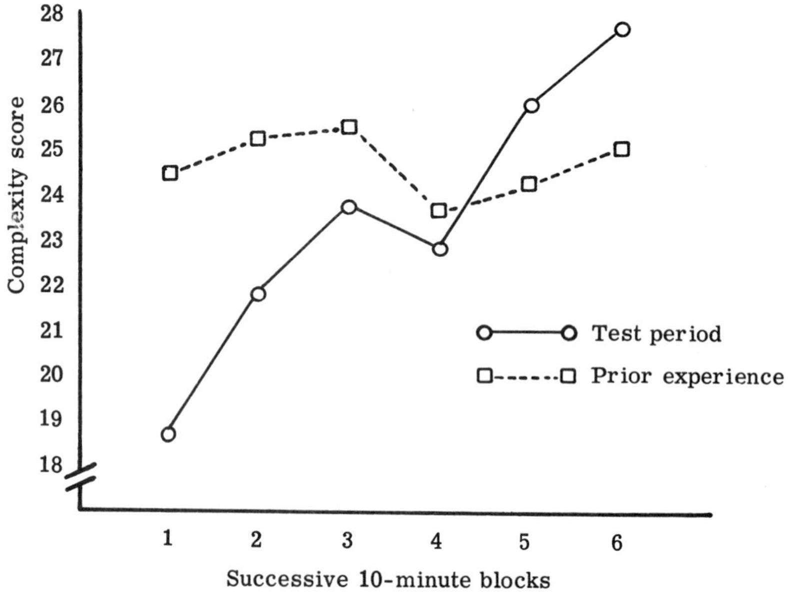

FIGURE 17. Changes in stimulus preference with time.

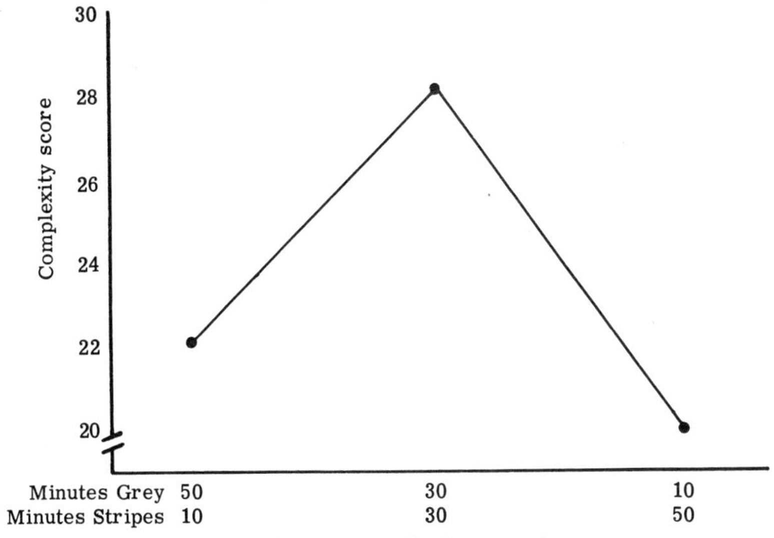

FIGURE 18. Generalized effects of stimulus exposure.

30 minutes and to the stripes for 30 minutes. The long exposure group was exposed to grey for ten minutes and to the stripes for 50 minutes.

At the end of the hour for each group, the 3/4-inch stripes were removed and the other four stripe patterns were introduced, one in each of the quadrants of the maze. The animals were then replaced, and their choices over a period of an hour were recorded. There were six animals in a group, a total of 18 in the experiment.

Complexity scores were again achieved by assigning arbitrary values to the stimuli ranging from a value of 1 to the widest stimulus pattern and a value of 4 to the narrowest. This value is then multiplied by the number of minutes in each ten-minute block spent in each compartment. The scores could thus range from a minimum of 10 to a maximum of 40.

FIGURE 17 shows the three groups combined to stress the progressive increase in preference for the more complex patterns over the hour of test compared to the exposure hour. FIGURE 18 replots the data to stress the differential effects of the exposure on the three groups.

The results are, in part, expected from complexity theory and, are in part, quite at variance with the expectation. During the one-hour test period, there is a progressive change in preference upward on the complexity dimension. The shift of nearly 10 points in FIGURE 17 indicates a shift of about one whole step across the "big" interval. In the first ten minutes the predominant preference was for the compartment with the 1 & 1/2-inch stripes, and in the last ten minutes, the predominant preference is for the compartment with the 3/8-inch stripes. This finding is in agreement with complexity theory.

The finding portrayed in FIGURE 18 is not easily explicable from the theory. The animals exposed to the 3/4-inch stripes for 30 minutes show a greater preference for more complex stimuli than does either the group exposed for ten minutes or the group exposed for 50 minutes. The locus of the problem may lie in small part in the wide gap between 3/8 inches and 1 & 1/2-inches, created when

TABLE 9

FIRST-ORDER TRANSITIONAL PROBABILITIES

		3 in.	1½ in.	⅜ in.	$\frac{3}{16}$ in.
		Short Exposure Group			
FROM	3 in.	.27	.03	.13	.07
	1½ in.	.00	.03	.03	.03
	⅜ in.	.13	.03	.10	.03
	$\frac{3}{16}$ in.	.00	.00	.07	.03
		Middle Exposure Group			
FROM	3 in.	.00	.00	.07	.03
	1½ in.	.00	.00	.03	.07
	⅜ in.	.00	.03	.13	.03
	$\frac{3}{16}$ in.	.03	.07	.00	.50
		Long Exposure Group			
FROM	3 in.	.27	.03	.17	.07
	1½ in.	.10	.10	.03	.03
	⅜ in.	.07	.07	.00	.00
	$\frac{3}{16}$ in.	.00	.00	.03	.03

the middle stimulus was used for exposure, but why the three groups should react to that gap as they did is not clear.

The first-order transitional probabilities for the three groups are contained in TABLE 9. If one compares the probabilities in the diagonals immediately adjacent to the main diagonal with the three values in each case in the lower left and upper right corners, there is some support for the "gap" theory. The outer corners show higher probabilities than the adjacent diagonals. This is the reverse of the finding in the previous Tables. It indicates a tendency to go from one extreme to the other, rather than from one stimulus to one that is adjacent on the *a priori* scale.

One might conclude from this analysis that the animals were not reacting to the stimuli as representing four values on a single dimension. However, since the progression from simple to complex is quite clear, one would argue from that evidence that they were reacting to the stimuli as if on a complexity scale. The only *post hoc* explanation that has emerged is that the gap creates a situation in which the animals react as if there were only two points on the scale, narrow and wide. A convincing resolution of this finding lies in the future.

Effect of Stimulus Range on Complexity and Preference¶¶

In the studies of judged complexity and preference in tartan patterns discussed earlier in this report, human subjects tended to respond to the range of stimuli presented to them. If they had a narrow range of stimuli on the less complex end of the scale, they tended to judge the upper end of their stimulus set as more complex than a group with the full range. If subjects judged only a set of more complex stimuli, they tended to judge the middle absolute range as less complex than subjects with the full range. From a variety of studies, it seemed possible that rats also responded to the range of stimuli presented to them rather than to responding on an absolute basis.

¶¶ This study was carried out by Wade Boykin as a masters level research project, 1968–1969. It resulted in a paper entitled The Effects of Level and Range of Complexity Values on Visual Preferences in Rats.

Boykin divided 18 (naive, male, Long Evans) rats at about 100–150 days of age into three groups of six animals each. One group (A) was to be exposed to a narrow range of relatively simple stimuli, a second group (B) was to be exposed to a narrow range of stimuli of high complexity, and a third group (C) was to be exposed to the full range. The stimuli selected on *a priori* grounds along with the items used with each of the three groups were the following:

		A	B	C
Simple end	2-inch horizontal stripes	X		X
	2-inch vertical stripes	X		
	4 checkers per 4 × 4 square	X		X
	9 checkers per 4 × 4 square	X		
	16 checkers per 4 × 4 square	X	X	X
	25 checkers per 4 × 4 square		X	
	49 checkers per 4 × 4 square		X	X
	81 checkers per 4 × 4 square		X	
Complex end	144 checkers per 4 × 4 square		X	X

The experimental apparatus was a circular device with a center compartment from which radiated six doors permitting access, from the center, to six equally sized truncated pie-shaped compartments. These compartment walls were lined with the stimuli.

There were six compartments and five stimuli. One compartment was utilized as an entrance compartment. When the animal left the entrance compartment, it was closed behind him so that he had access during the trial to five stimulus compartments and the central compartment.

A trial consisted of ten minutes in the maze for 12 consecutive days for each animal.

The behavior of the animal was recorded on six of the channels of an Esterline-Angus recorder by marking where the animal was at all times during the trial as it activated the appropriate event marker.

FIGURE 19 shows the total amount of time spent by each group in each of

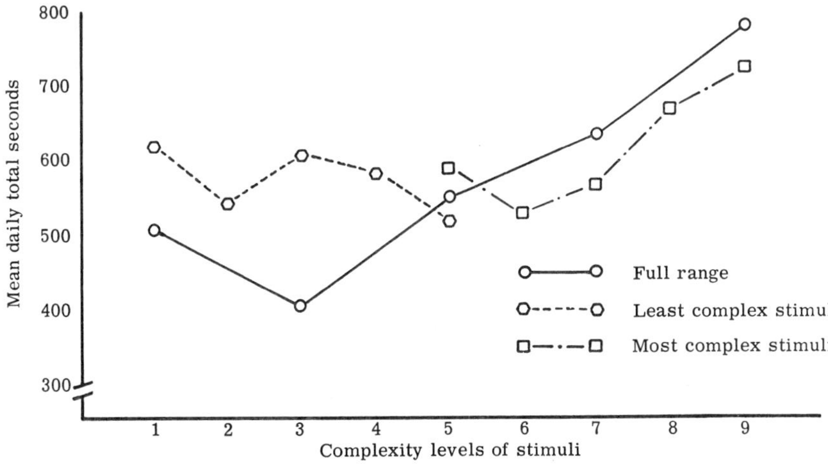

FIGURE 19—The effect of stimulus range on preference.

the available stimulus compartments. Those in the low range of complexities do not show a preference. Those in the higher range show some preference for the more complex stimuli. The group exposed to the full range show a definite preference for the more complex stimuli. Thus the range of stimuli available did have an effect. Preference was more clearly expressed with the wider range of stimuli.

Frequency versus Duration of Response as a Function of Stimulus

When a set of stimuli is available for choice in the sense that the organism can see all the stimuli and choose among them, it is difficult to separate the effects of complexity on the frequency of choice from the effects on duration of choice. The necessity of distinguishing the factors determining the termination of a response from those that govern the next choice has been pointed out elsewhere.[7] The concept of action decrement[6] can be used to account for the termination of a response. Stimulus complexity may be a factor in delaying termination and, thus, in controlling the duration. Optimal stimulus levels should produce the maximum duration, and stimuli either more or less than optimum should produce shorter durations.

A test of this possibility has been devised by Stephen Sales.[5] He constructed a box that consisted of a compartment that was about a foot in each dimension and that was totally dark when the lid was in place. On one side of the box there was a small hole through which a rat was able to stick his head far enough to break a photoelectric cell beam, thus allowing itself to see what was in the adjacent compartment. The adjacent compartment was arranged with a translucent panel positioned about 5 inches from the hole at floor level and slanted slightly toward the animal at the top. This panel was backlighted. The photoelectric cell was used to record the behavior of the rat.

The panel was replaceable. Stimulus complexity was varied by constructing nine such panels. Each consisted of a checkered pattern and they differed in the number of elements 2, 4, 9, 16, 25, 64, 100, 196, and 256.

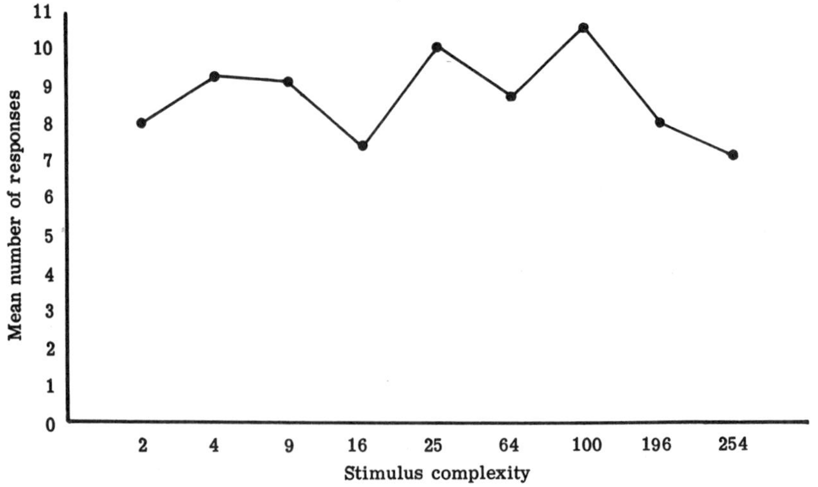

FIGURE 20. Frequency of response as a function of stimulus complexity.

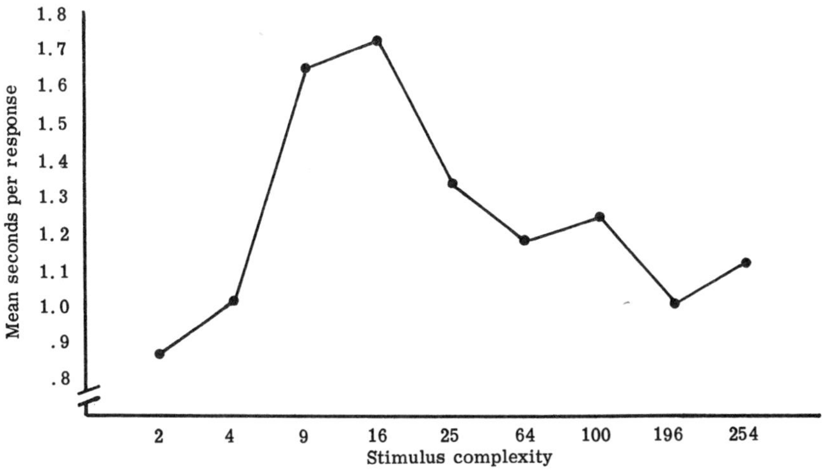

FIGURE 21. Duration of response as a function of stimulus complexity.

Nine groups of 15 rats each (total 135, 108 male and 27 female) were each handled extensively and then introduced individually into the box. Ten seconds after introduction, the light was turned on in the adjacent compartment. Each animal was left in the box for a total of eight minutes. Each animal was tested only once and with a single stimulus.

The photocell recorded the frequency of response through a counter, and the total duration of responding through a clock that accumulated the total amount of time the animal's head was in a position to break the photobeam.

FIGURE 20 shows the frequency of responding in the nine groups thus self-exposed to the nine levels of stimulus complexity. There appears to be no orderly relationship between complexity and frequency. This result might be expected, since the animal could not see the stimulus until he responded.

FIGURE 21 shows the average duration of the responses, calculated by dividing the total response time by the frequency. Here, there is a clear optimum with stimuli around 9 and 16 elements. Thus, the complexity of the stimulus affected the duration of the response, with optimum complexity producing the longer responses, and either simpler or more complex stimuli producing responses of lesser durations.

Summary of Animal Studies of Complexity and Preference

The major finding of the animal studies of complexity and preference is that animals do tend to show preferences for stimuli of progressively increasing complexity with increased exposure in the choice situation. A correlated finding is that when the animal could not see the stimulus until he made a response, stimulus complexity increased the duration of the response. This finding is interesting in a context in which it is important to distinguish between factors that affect the termination of a psychological event and those that affect the choice of the next event.

Analysis of sequences of responses permitted the scaling of disparate stimuli and confirmed the fact that the animals were indeed responding to the order of the stimuli along a complexity scale. Animals were found to respond to the range of stimuli available, as had been found in the human studies. An attempt to demonstrate the predicted effect of prior exposure to a stimulus on a complexity dimension on subsequent choices yielded clear, but inexplicable, results.

References

1. Berlyne, D. E. 1960. Conflict, Arousal and Curiosity. McGraw-Hill. New York.
2. Dember, W. N. 1960. The Psychology of Perception. Henry Holt and Co. New York.
3. Hebb, D. O. 1949. The Organization of Behavior. John Wiley and Sons, Inc. New York.
4. Innes, T. 1938. The Tartan of the Clans and Families of Scotland. Johnston. Edinburg and London.
5. Sales, S. M. 1968. Stimulus complexity as a determinant of approach behavior and inspection time in the hooded rat. Canad. J. Psychol./Rev. Canad. Psychol. **22:** 11–17.
6. Walker, E. L. 1958. Action decrement and its relation to learning. Psychol. Rev. **65:** 129–142.
7. Walker, E. L. 1964. Psychological complexity as a basis of a theory of motivation and choice. *In* Nebraska Symposium on Motivation. Levine, D., Ed. University of Nebraska Press. Lincoln, Neb.
8. Walker, E. L. & B. E. Walker. 1964. Response to stimulus complexity in the rat. Psychol. Rec. **14:** 489–497.

Discussion

Sydney Vernon (*Willimantic, Conn.*): Dr. Walker indicated that art students accepted a greater degree of complexity than history and law students. I venture to submit that since these stimuli were visual, the art students had greater skills, and possibly, if the stimuli had been auditory, the history students might have accepted greater complexity, and if the stimuli had to do with social or interpersonal relationships, maybe your law students would have done better. Dr. Walker also indicated that certain sets of stimuli were satisfying. Now this implies a visceral reaction, and I submit that the whole perceptive mechanism doesn't involve merely the central nervous system, but comes from a combination of mind and body. To extend the concept that mind and body are part of the perceptive mechanism, I'd like to refer to the simple example of ulcers. Here, the flood of stimuli in the person who has ulcers gets to the brain, jumps over into his vegas, stimulates the stomach, pours out hydrochloric acid, and digests his mucosa.

The term "noise" was used, which always bothers me in scientific discussion. It seems to me that what is noise to one person may not be to another. The absence of noise means that the stimuli were meaningful, and if the stimuli were not meaningful, well then we use the term "noise." Of course I'm not speaking of the tremendous number of decibels that assail our accoustic organs, but, rather, scientifically. In his experiments with mice, and in dealing with the problem of assigning values to their peculiar behavior, Dr. Walker indicated that in those compartments that had colors, the grey, the stripes, and the checkered, the mice had a tendency to congregate in the grey area, and I submit that they did it because they felt secure there. Then later on the mice seemed to choose the battle area more and I submit that that was one time where they wanted privacy more than anything. Of course, all living creatures want to feel safe and want to feel important. Among other desires, they want variety, and that's why I think some of the mice stuck their heads through those holes.

And the degree of curiosity, or vitality, that Dr. Walker indicated the mice had possibly had something to do with the length of time they held their heads through those holes.

Dr. Walker: Well, let me try to respond to your comments. Concerning the experiment having to do with experience, I agree with you. I apparently didn't make myself clear in trying to shorten this. The point I was trying to make with respect to the experience of the art students was that it did have precisely the effect that you suggest. Because they had had more experience with visual stimuli, they were chosen. The law students were chosen because they had had less experience with visual stimuli. There were differences in the way in which they rated complexity, which was a result of their experience. While the data did not statistically demonstrate the optimal complexity shift upward for those subjects, it did demonstrate that they did react differently to the stimuli along the dimension that we were working with.

Now I should not have used the word noise. I was using it in the sense of "variance or error," a term that is referred to as "noise." This is not in my paper. In addition, I don't think I'll quibble with you over the language you choose to use with respect to the subject seeking that stimulus which represents his optimal complexity value. When you retranslate it, you use the word "security." This is acceptable. I used the word "preference."

Dr. Moore (*Brookdale Hospital*): There's been a great deal of work on complexity and creativity complexity, and intelligence complexity, and neuroticism. The material you presented seems to undercut the idea of individual differences in complexity and preference. Could you comment on this?

Dr. Walker: My experiments are not intended to undercut that idea. As a matter of fact, I think there are enormous individual differences. What we're trying to do is find the major dimension of individual differences. And this is the reason for the distinction between stimulus complexity and/or psychological complexity, where the individual's reaction is expected to be different. That is why, in all these studies, even with the rats, we try to carry out the study in such a manner that you can analyze the data of an individual subject independently of the others. And had we had time, I could have shown you that there were indeed individual difference in rats, one of which Rat Y, scaled those four stimuli differently from the other two that did. I feel that this is the major focus of the theory. Trying to find a way to dimensionalize, get your hands on a major dimension which does describe individual differences.

THE PERCEPTION OF GESTALT—1969

Harry Helson, Ph.D.
University of Massachusetts, Amherst, Mass.

Gestalt psychology made the study of forms, wholes, segregated units, and connected processes a fruitful and legitimate object of scientific psychology. The perception of objects like trees, pictures, tables, and human faces had been banished as such from psychology both by thc Wundt-Müller-Titchener school of introspection and by the Brentano school of Akt psychology. The former reduced perception to complexes of sensations and images that were meaningless in themselves, while the latter admitted only psychic acts, and not their intended objects, as the proper subjects of study. To establish the fundamental nature of perceived objects and events. Gestalt psychologists made the concept of organization the basic postulate of their system. Organization, according to them, is immediately intuited and automatically achieved through dynamical self-distribution of processes in the nervous system.[1]

Granting the great contributions of Gestalt psychology, it would be surprising if advances had not been made during the last half century since Wertheimer's famous 1912[2] paper advancing the Gestalt theory of form perception. We can now envisage organization as part of the broader problem of the formation of classes,[3] not only perceptual but cognitive and emotional, and also as a manifestation of the organism's adaptations to its environment. As an example of the need for a broader theory to encompass Gestalt phenomena, consider the remark made by an eight-year-old girl on a walk in the country as she puzzled over something she saw: "Is that a small tree or a large bush?" In the one class it was small; in the other, large. While the Gestalt psychologists were content to ascribe such phenomena merely to differences in organization, we must ask how and why the same object may be perceived with different properties in different contexts or by different individuals in the same context. To this and similar problems I will return later in this paper.

According to the position presented here, an adequate theory of perceptual organization must take into account not only contextual and background stimuli but also residual stimuli from past experience that influence given stimuli. Provision must be made for anchoring or predominant stimuli that are made so by such factors as intensity, size, frequency or because they have special claims due to familiarity, ego-involvement, and the like. The Gestalt concept of interaction is subsumed to our concept of pooling by which adaptation levels (AL) are formed. According to this view *all* conditions of stimulation tend to pool in forming levels. Often it is forgotten that order of presentation, timing, spacing, and many other apparently "neutral" aspects in the environment may have decisive effects on AL by pooling with the more obvious factors usually studied experimentally. Finally, an adequate theory of perceptual organization must be capable of quantitative formulation, and the concept of the AL as the behavioral zero with its underlying physiological equilibrium meets this requirement. Adaptation level, defined as a weighted log mean of focal, background, and residual stimuli, allows behavioral zero to vary as either or both stimulus and organismic factors change. The concept of AL is not restricted to sensory-perceptual data for it has been applied to cognitive (verbal), affective, and motivational states also.[3] In the remainder of this paper I shall show how AL theory has succeeded in concretizing and quantifying perception of Gestalt and related problems.

There are many facets of Gestalt theory that we might single out for consideration, but I shall limit myself to some advances that have been made in the treatment and theory of organized wholes in several realms of behavior. Limits of time and space do not permit consideration of approaches such as information theory, decision theory, and theory of signal detection, which have proved fruitful in the study of perception, judgment, and discriminal processes. I shall emphasize particularly advances in analyzing and quantifying some Gestalt phenomena in perception, cognition, learning, and judgment. According to the Gestalt point of view, properties of organized wholes are lost if they are subjected to analysis and this was certainly true of the introspective analysis current at the time their movement was born. But there are different kinds of analysis. In later years Gestalt psychologists admitted that there could be "good" types of analysis if they dealt with natural parts of wholes as opposed to the artificial parts of introspection. Instead of asking observers to analyze their perceptions, as was the practice in Titchener's laboratory at Cornell, we now call for reports on observed phenomena as we vary conditions of stimulation. In the method of single stimuli or absolute judgment, we do not even ask observers to compare variables with a standard, as we now know from adaptation-level considerations that the presence of the standard exerts a predominant influence on prevailing level and thereby affects the report of the stimulus variable under consideration. The way in which perceptual wholes are preserved while being analyzed and measured can best be shown by a concrete example.

In a recent study of an illusion of extent wherein the perceived length of a line is influenced by the size (area) of boxes tangent to its ends, Restle and Merryman[4] employed the following technique of investigation. Observers were presented lines of 4, 6, 8, 10, 12, and 14 units in length with boxes of either 4, 6, 8, 10, 12, or 14 units on a side. Observers were merely asked to denote the apparent length of the center line by pressing one of six keys in which the extreme left key meant "quite short" and the extreme right key "quite long," while the intermediate keys denoted intermediate lengths. The results show that the larger the box size, the shorter the center line appears for each line length except the two shortest lines of 4 and 6 units. Our interest in this problem extends beyond the phenomenological data merely relating perceived lengths of lines and box sizes. The analysis employed by Restle and Merryman makes possible evaluation of the contributions of the parts of the stimulus configuration and of the organism to the total perception. Assuming that the apparent length of the center line is a function of its own length, the size of the boxes, and residual factors within the organism, Restle and Merryman, using a simple linear hypothesis, write the following equation:

$$J_A = L/A \qquad (1)$$

where J_A is the judged length of center line L, and A, the adaptation level, is a weighted mean of line length, box size, and residuals as follows:

$$A = (L^p B^q R^r)^{1/p+q+r} \qquad (2)$$

where L has the same meaning as above, B is box size in linear units, and R denotes residual factors mainly in the organism, and p, q, and r are weighting coefficients that can be normalized. The exponent in Equation 2 then becomes 1 and we can now rewrite Equation 1 as follows by substituting the value of A from Equation 2:

$$J_A = L/A = L^{1-p} B^{-q} R^{-r} \qquad (3)$$

The least squares solution for the values of the weighting coefficients turn out to be 0.082 for line length, 0.138 for box size, and 0.593 for the residual factors. (We will not consider here the reason why the sum of the weighting coefficients does not equal 1). Thus box size is more important than line length, and residuals are more important than the other two factors in determining the magnitude of the illusion. It is noteworthy that the largest contribution to the illusion is by the organism and this argues against a wholly autonomous determination of Gestalt properties. The illusion depends upon organismic as well as configurational factors. The AL model thus makes possible analysis and evaluation of the various components in the total perception and provides for the integral role of the organism in perception of Gestalt.

That the past and present state of the organism must be taken into account in perception of Gestalt hardly needs elaboration, yet its experimental demonstration is important in view of the emphasis on purely stimulus factors by the Gestalt psychologists. Adaptation-level theory takes into account the role of prior adaptations in phenomenal structuration in a way not envisaged in classical *Gestalt theorie.* Thus Bell and Bevan[5] showed that Wertheimer's law of grouping, which says that the form of grouping is most natural which involves the smallest interval between elements, must be qualified, for when observers were previously exposed to a matrix of dots organized as rows (or colmuns), they reported columns (or rows) more frequently than did control group without the previous experience of distinct rows or columns. Similarly, what was perceived as cases of good continuation, similarity, and closure was a function of previous experience. We cannot neglect the strong influence of predominant stimuli, anchors or backgrounds on perceived organization.

Owing to their rejection of introspective analyses in terms of sensory attributes, the Gestalt psychologists failed to recognize how important such dimensional factors as intensity, time, area, quality, frequency, and other conditions of stimulation can be in perception of Gestalt. Furthermore their preoccupation with stable visual patterns resulted in overlooking the importance of intra-organismic norms in perception. We have seen, in the study by Bell and Bevan[5] just cited, that even stable spatial configurations are affected by previous adaptations, and it is easy to show that variation in a dimensional attribute of even a single stimulus in a series results in different judgments of the series as a whole. Thus in a study by Helson and Kozaki[6] in which observers were asked to judge sizes of squares 36, 45, 54, 63, and 72 mm on a side on a nine-point rating scale ranging from very, very small through medium to very, very large, when the largest square was exposed for 1.0 second while the others were exposed for only 0.20 second, the judgments were all depressed, i.e., the squares were judged smaller than by a control group in which all the squares were exposed at the same time, viz., 0.20 second, as shown in FIGURE 1. In the case of another group when the smallest square was exposed for a longer time than the others, the judgments of the squares shifted upward to a significant extent, as is also seen in FIGURE 1. Here a dimensional variation in only one of a series of five stimuli results in altered perception of the sizes of all the stimuli.

Configurational principles, when applied to perceptual learning, must be modified to include qualitative and organismic factors, as shown in a study of transposition of a lightness discrimination by Helson and Kaplan.[7] In this study, which was a replication with some modifications of Köhler's study with chimpanzees, subjects were shown a series of five gray squares having reflectances of 15, 20, 28, 50, and 62 percent. These were arranged in random order on a

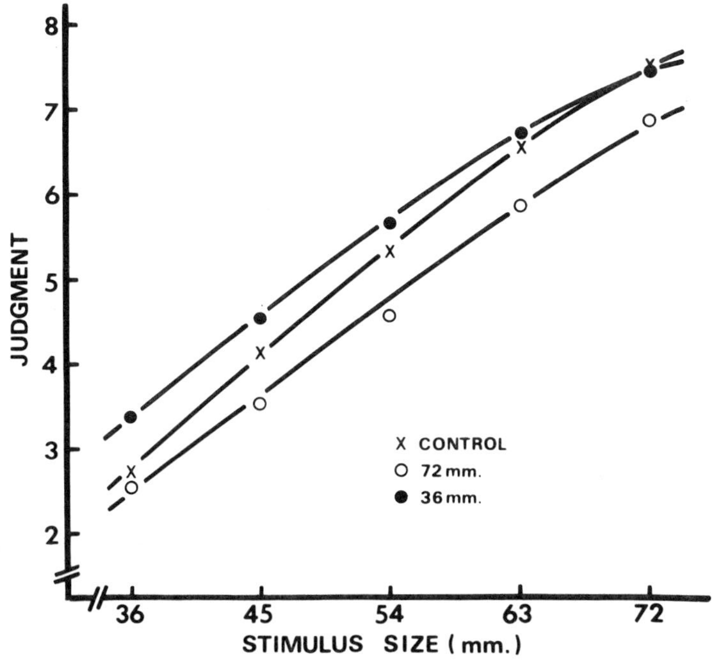

FIGURE 1. This shows that longer duration of the largest stimulus (72 mm) causes a downward shift in judgments of size of the other series stimuli, while longer duration of the smallest stimulus (36 mm) causes an upward shift in the judgments.

black background. The subjects were simply asked to choose one, and if they chose the square of middle lightness, they were either reinforced by being told "correct," or otherwise, told "wrong." After ten correct choices of the middle gray stimulus, the subjects were then shown the same grays on a white background arranged in random order and asked to choose one. According to both the Gestalt prediction and the elementaristic theories rejected by Köhler, the same stimulus should be chosen on the white background that was chosen on the black background because according to the former, it was still the middle stimulus, and because according to the latter, it was the identical stimulus. According to the theory I am espousing, subjects should choose a gray having the same relation to prevailing adaptation level on the white background that the training stimulus had to its adaptation level on black background. Since the adaptation level was raised on white background, subjects should choose a gray of higher reflectance than that on which they were trained, for the one on which they were trained was above AL, and it required a stimulus of higher reflectance to be above AL on white background. Two stimuli having 50% and 62% reflectance had about the same lightness on white background as the 28% reflectance had on black background and these were predicted to be the ones chosen. Sixty-one percent of the 62 subjects did indeed choose one of these grays, with only 32% of the subjects choosing the training gray. An almost identical experiment was performed independently by Campbell and Kral[8] with parakeets as subjects. The six birds responded on the transfer trials with 85, 80, 70, 85, 90, and 45 percent choices according to AL theory. Their average performance, 76 percent choices of lighter stimulus on white background, was even more in accord with AL theory than the human results, probably because Campbell and Kral used 20, instead of only one, transposition trials. Even more striking transfer results were found by Capehart and Pease[9] who used a somewhat different design, employing lifted weights as stimuli.

We can now return to the problem of perception as part of the broader problem of cognitive systems. It is almost a truism to say that conception enters into every perception and that even the simplest sensory process has a cognitive component. William James[10] recognized this when he pointed out that every sensation carries some knowledge with it. We perceive objects not merely as segregated units in the sense of that used by Gestalt psychologists but as members of classes. We see a man not only as figured against a background but also as a short or tall man, stout or thin, white or black, bright or dull, kind or cruel. I do not mean by these dichotomies to imply that we perceive only extremes–far from it. Every object is perceived and judged according to internal norms, adaptation levels, operating quite automatically for the most part, but sometimes according to explicit criteria. Fine as well as gross discriminations and judgments are made with respect to prevailing norms. The same object may be classed in one way at one time, in another at another time, depending upon the effective norm of the moment. Thus individual differences, differences in one individual's responses to the same stimulus, and the same response to different stimuli receive explanation from a single set of assumptions. The concept of changing level provides a solid basis for the relativity of judgment stressed by psychologists from the beginning of modern experimental psychology in the last century to the present.

As an example of the operation of AL in cognitive organization, let us consider some results of an experiment by Helson and Kozaki.[11] Observers judged the sizes of ten squares ranging from 20 to 150 mm on a side in terms of a rating scale ranging from very, very small through medium to very, very large. Five of the squares were colored green and five were colored orange. The green squares were 20, 27, 36, 48, and 64 mm on a side; the orange squares were 48, 64, 84, 110, and 110 mm on a side. It is thus evident that two squares were in both the small green and large orange series. The squares were presented in random order, yet the average judgments of the observers plotted in FIGURE 2 show that they were ordered into two classes on the basis of their colors. Not only are the slopes of the fitted curves for the green and orange judgments significantly different, but the two squares common to the two sets are also judged significantly different: the 48- and 64-mm squares are judged larger in the green series than are the same squares in the orange series. After our experiment was completed, we discovered that a similar experiment had been made by Brown and McBride[12] at the University of California at Berkeley a dozen or more years ago but with lifted weights as the stimuli. In their experiment subjects judged a series of weights 200, 300, 400, 500, and 600 g colored green and another series 500, 600, 700, 800, and 900 g colored red. Thus the 500- and 600-g weights were common to the two series. After several rounds of judgments, the subjects were asked to judge a test weight of 550 g both when it was red and when it was green. As in our experiment the test weight was judged greater (heavier) when green, i.e., when at the top of the series, than when red, i.e., at the bottom of the series. In discussing this experiment, the late Professor Köhler[13] attributed the difference in judgment of the test weight to the fact that it belonged to different organizations when differently colored.

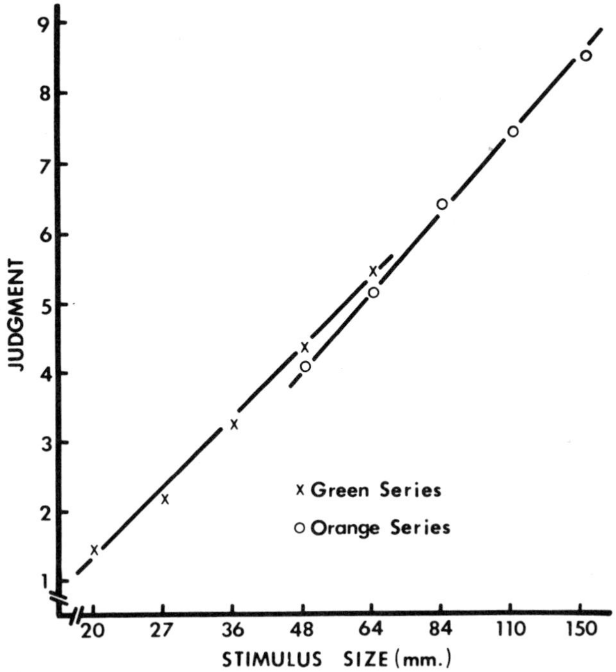

FIGURE 2. This shows that the same stimuli (48 and 64 mm) are judged differently when above the adaptation level in the green series and below the adaptation level in the orange series. Note that the slopes of the curves for green and orange series are significantly different also.

We cannot rest content, however, with an explanation that merely ascribes observed effects to differences in organization. We must ask why the differently colored squares and weights were differently organized in the two experiments. We know that objects are grouped into classes depending on their relations to prevailing AL. In the green series the common weight and the common squares are *above* AL and are therefore judged above medium (heavy; large) while in the other color they are *below* AL and are therefore judged below medium (light; small). Furthermore, AL theory provides a quantitative treatment that enables us to determine how heavy or large a stimulus will be judged once the value of AL and the stimulus-judgment function are known, something that is not possible from a purely phenomenological concept of organization.

The way in which anchors exert a predominant influence on organization was also shown in the same study.[11] Three groups of six subjects each were presented sets of red and green squares, 36, 45, 54, 63, and 72 mm on a side, in random order, to be judged for size as in the first part of the study. With one group, each of the judged stimuli was preceded by a red square 90 mm on a side serving as a large anchor; another group was given a small red anchor 18 mm on a side. A third group acted as controls by judging the stimuli without interpolated anchors. As seen from FIGURE 3, the large red anchor depressed the judgments of the red stimuli to a significantly greater extent than those of the green stimuli, and the small red anchor raised the judgments of the red squares significantly more than of the green squares. While the judgments of both the red and green sets of stimuli were significantly affected by the large and small anchors, as shown in FIGURE 3 by comparing their curves with the curve of the controls, the differential, selective action of the anchors on stimuli of the same color is unmistakable. These results were replicated with two other groups given green anchors. In this case the curves for red and green stimuli reversed because the green judgments shifted more than the red. A fuller account of this study will appear in another publication.

At this point it should be noted that another advance in the treatment of factors influencing organization has been made regarding effects of subliminal stimulation. Subliminal stimulation offers special problems for Gestalt theory because, being present, its influence on perceived data cannot be ascribed to traces, yet it is not phenomenologically given and does not appear as part of the perceptual field. Studies by a number of workers have shown that effects of subliminal stimulation pool with supraliminal stimuli to influence adaptation levels and thus the organization of the perceived field (Bevan & Pritchard[14] with sound stimuli; Black & Bevan[15] with shock; Boardman & Goldstone[16] with visual size). Similarly, pooling across different sense modalities, showing that interaction is even more widespread than envisaged in classical Gestalt theory, has also been investigated within the framework of AL theory.[17–19]

Sufficient evidence has now accumulated from many experimental investigations to warrant some generalizations applicable to more complex life situations than are possible in laboratory approaches. First, the operation of internal norms

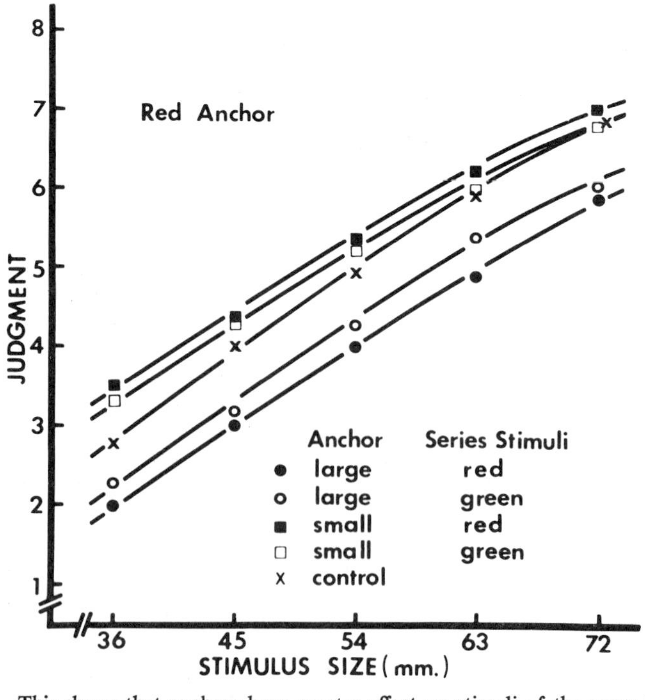

FIGURE 3. This shows that anchors have greater effect on stimuli of the same (red) color than on stimuli of another (green) color.

is ubiquitous: all behavior is referable to prevailing adaptations. Such norms may be implicit or explicit. They are the result of all the input to which organisms have been exposed including contextual and subliminal stimuli. A single intense or significant experience or mild, repeated stimulation may have profound influence on prevailing level. If our assumption that all behavior is referable to prevailing AL is correct, then it follows that *there can be no change in behavior without change in internal norms*. Internal norms may be changed by varying input (focal and/or background stimuli) and by change in residuals or the adaptations already in existence. But we can modify residuals only by modifying present situations and so we are led back to variation of input as the primary source of behavior modification. However, the recognition that inner norms must be modified before there can be a change in outer behavior is in itself a step toward understanding the mechanisms of character formation.

Results of investigations of anchor effects are not mere analogs of complex socioeconomic forces at work in our society. Just as judgment of a single stimulus is influenced by other stimuli and, especially, by contrasting anchors, so the perception of a group's situation, its expectations, hopes, and aspirations are determined not only by its own standard of living but also by what it perceives to be the condition of other groups in the society. We venture the hypothesis that much of the unrest in our society in recent years springs as much, and possibly more, from the contrast of life in the slums with life in the better parts of our cities and suburbs. Those on a subsistence level of living ask why a government that can spend billions on a far-off war cannot move faster in the eradication of slums; why a nation that can spend enough money to dig a hole in the ground for military purposes (which was abandoned before even being used) could not have allocated this sum, which was large enough to support a nearby impoverished school district for 100 or more years! While the poor have always been with us, the *contrast* of superabundance in some segments of our society with poverty next door, and the contrast of spending billions for the military while cutting funds for schools, hospitals, and medical research are recent manifestations of a society in disequilibrium. We must learn to mitigate these sharp contrasts if we are to survive as a democracy.

The contrasts that are stirring masses of citizens are heightened by modern media of communication. People perceive from TV and radio, from movies and stage plays, from books and articles, and from the daily newspaper, the conditions of life in various strata of our society, the operation of our government, the way in which our courts and law enforcement agencies function, and the fighting of a far-off war. All of this constitutes the input that determines the norms governing people's lives. What we perceive is of primary importance in how we behave and how we perceive is referable to our internal norms. These must be included in the theory of Gestalt perception today.

References

1. Helson, H. 1925 & 1926. The psychology of Gestalt. Amer. J. Psychol. **36:** 342–370; 494–526; **37:** 25–62; 189–216.
2. Wertheimer, M. 1912. Experimentelle Studien über das Sehen von Bewegung. Zeitschrift für Psychologie **61:** 161–278.
3. Helson, H. 1964. Adaptation-Level Theory. Harper and Row. New York, N. Y.
4. Restle, F. & C. T. Merryman. 1968. An adaptation-level theory account of a relative-size illusion. Psychon. Sci. **12:** 229–230.
5. Bell, R. A. & W. Bevan. 1968. Influence of anchors upon the operation of certain Gestalt organizing principles. J. Exper. Psychol. **78:** 670–678.

6. HELSON, H. & T. KOZAKI. 1968. Effects of duration of series and anchor-stimuli on judgments of perceived size. Amer. J. Psychol. **81**: 291–302.
7. HELSON, H. & S. KAPLAN. Unpublished study described more fully in Reference 5 above.
8. CAMPBELL, D. T. & T. P. KRAL. 1958. Transposition away from a rewarded stimulus card to a non-rewarded one as a function of a shift in background. J. Compar. Physiol. Psychol. **51**: 592–595.
9. CAPEHART, J. & V. PEASE. 1968. An application of adaptation-level theory to transposition responses in a conditional discrimination. Psychon. Sci. **10**: 147–148.
10. JAMES, W. 1890. Principles of Psychology. Vol. II, 3ff. Henry Holt and Co. New York, N. Y.
11. HELSON, H. & T. KOZAKI. Unpublished study.
12. BROWN, D. & P. MCBRIDE. Personal communication.
13. KÖHLER, W. 1966–67. Unpublished lecture delivered at Dartmouth College and personally communicated to Lloyd Avant.
14. BEVAN, W. & J. F. PRITCHARD. 1963. Effect of "subliminal" tones upon the judgment of loudness. J. Exper. Psychol. **66**: 23–29.
15. BLACK, R. W. & W. BEVAN. 1960. The effect of subliminal shock upon the judged intensity of weak shock. Amer. J. Psychol. **73**: 262–267.
16. BOARDMAN, W. K. & S. GOLDSTONE. 1962. Effects of subliminal anchors upon judgments of size. Perceptual and Motor Skills **14**: 475–482.
17. BEHAR, I. & W. BEVAN. 1961. The perceived duration of auditory and visual intervals: cross-modal comparison and interaction. Amer. J. Psychol. **74**: 17–26.
18. BEVAN, W. & J. F. PRITCHARD. 1964. The effect of visual intensities upon the judgment of loudness. Amer. J. Psychol. **77**: 93–98.
19. GOLDSTONE, S., W. K. BOARDMAN & W. T. LHAMON. 1959. Intersensory comparison of temporal judgments. Amer. J. Psychol. **57**: 243–248.

Discussion

DR. SYDNEY VERNON: Could Dr. Helson give us a definition of a Gestalt? I'm interested also in his description, in his defining the term "adaptation," because I find that he described a stiuation in which adaptation went up and judgment went down. I think this applies to the present social situation described in some detail in his concluding remarks. I think that there are a tremendous number of people who are trying to adapt to an unpleasant situation, and yet, their judgment is perhaps going down. I would also like a definition of "internal norms." I noted that in the description, he did indicate that the gestalt process, which involves sensory, perceptive, and cognitive factors, was an intuitive and also a behavior process. This indicates that perception is not merely a sensory experience, but is also a reactive experience, which perhaps fortifies the speculation that we don't think merely with our brain, but with our whole body. And certainly when he says that repetitive advertising becomes unpleasant, I think he indicates, too, that the body is involved. I venture the hypothesis that one reason why repetition becomes upleasant is that a certain set of nerve cells becomes fatigued; they become refractory. They use up so much oxygen in metabolism that they are finally reduced to an anaerobic type of metabolism, that there is a certain amount of cellular acidosis in some cells; they become painful and that's why repetition is unpleasant. And further, in connection with the orange and the green, I've watched airplanes at night and I've noticed that, even though the candle power of the red and green lights must be equal, one of them seems bigger than the other. I wonder whether this is something that biophysicists will have to explain to us. After all, there is a chemical reaction involved, visual purple or rhodopsin is consumed, and it's a possibility that there is a differential or quantitative consumption of this chemical material, in accordance with the different colors.

DR. HELSON: Regarding the first question, I just define the Gestalt as any segregated unit in the field. I have already defined the adaptation level using a simple formula here.

DR. VERNON: It is mathematics then.

DR. HELSON: Yes.

DR. VERNON: What are internal norms?

DR. HELSON: They're adaptation levels.

DR. VERNON: Well, then do you think that a Gestalt reaction is also a response?

DR. HELSON: I think a reaction is a response, yes, using your terminology.

JOHN F. CORSO (*State University of New York*): Would Dr. Helson care to comment on the matter of changing adaptation level as it might relate to the shift in preference for more complex stimuli, such as those pointed out in Doctor Walker's paper?

DR. HELSON: Yes, while I was listening to his paper, I was thinking of some of the AL possibilities there, and of course there is no better illustration of changes in adaptation levels than the history of music, the history of painting, and the arts in general. I think the history of music lends beautiful support to Dr. Walker's position. The ancients, and medievalists liked what we consider to be the soft fusions, fifths and octaves. Then we had the period in which thirds and sixths were preferred, in which the elements stand out more, and you have a less unified auditory gestalt. It's more complex. And now we're in an age when we're getting to like seconds and sevenths. And I think the same holds in the history of painting too. I am bewildered by the complexity of a lot of modern abstract art as compared with the classical representational art. And I think Dr. Walker's studies get beautiful support from the history of the arts.

CHARLES HARRIS (*Bell Telephone Laboratories*): In your talk you emphasized experiments that involved rating on a six- or seven-point scale and so on. I'm sure that in the case of brightness, or illusion of line length, you would get similar results if you estimated in inches in the case of line length or in that of brightness, estimated on some absolute scale of brightness. What I'm wondering about is whether experiments like that have been done with the green and red series, either by rating with some kind of units of size, or for example, trying to match the sizes of the reds and the greens?

DR. HELSON: I published a study in Perception and Psychophysics about a year ago with Aiko Kozaki in which the estimates of dot patterns were in numbers. And we got even bigger anchor effects than we did with the rating scale. Look up Helson and Kozaki in Perception and Psychophysics.

PART II. PERCEPTION OF THE INNER WORLD

INNER PERCEPTION IN TERMS OF DEPTH PSYCHOLOGY

Joseph L. Henderson, M.D.
Stanford University Hospital Medical School
San Francisco, Calif.

The perennial philosophy in all ages and at all times has maintained the belief that there is an inner objective world, just as there is an outer objective world. Neoplatonists spoke of being in touch with a world soul or divine spirit from which man has fallen into this imperfect world to suffer and eventually, perhaps, return to our original state of grace. Zen Buddhists advised their followers to seek release through an experience of enlightenment called *Satori,* similar to the Hindu conception called *Samadhi.* These are religiously cultivated and highly disciplined perceptions of the inner world. But in the West, especially the modern West, following John Locke and the French philosopher-psychologists from the 17th century to our own, the conscious mind was thought to exist without history and without inner content, merely reflecting whatever excites interest from outer environment, all of which in the 18th century created an intellectual movement called the Enlightenment.

The one-sidedness of this Western viewpoint activated, in due course, a growing doubt as to its validity and this resulted in a rediscovery of that inner world which cannot be accounted for by the rational mind. It came to be called the "unconscious," with its own separate life and its own intrinsic meaning. The latter is not merely a distorted version of the rational daylight thoughts; it records the unconscious stages out of which consciousness gradually emerges. An excellent account of this development before the advent of modern depth psychology is found in L. L. Whyte's The Unconscious Before Freud.[1] All I can do in a brief paper is to give some account of a later stage since and including some of Freud's work, together with that of the neofreudian revisionists and especially the work of Jung. Jung was the first to suggest a term more in keeping with contemporary thinking than could be implied by the term the unconscious. He used the term, the "objective psyche," which combines both conscious and unconscious elements to reveal the inner contents of the psyche in a new way.

What depth psychology may be said to contribute that is different from previous studies, whether of philosophers or experimental psychologists, lies in describing: (1) The psychological function by which inner perceptions are made; and (2) The inner contents of the psyche, namely, that which can be perceived. I therefore propose to discuss my subject under these two headings, function and content.

The Psychological Function of Inner Perception

At an earlier time, the ego was regarded as a perceiving subject that functions as if it were an object, and this became an intellectual contradiction. We still speak of a strong or a weak ego as a thing we could measure or weigh, and its function is frequently discussed as if it were as mechanically constructed as a clock. This type of thinking stems from that same old psychological thinking dating from the 17th century, when de la Mettrie, for instance, maintained that the mind has thinking muscles as the body has walking muscles, which can be relaxed or tensed at will. This mechanistic attitude influenced psychoanalysis and even some of Jung's early work, but has at last been replaced in modern depth psychology (with reinforcement from psychobiology), by an organismic or "holistic" view of the ego function arising from "the experiencing person himself, both in his wholeness and uniqueness."[2] Accordingly, the ego, as an object for investigation, has in modern depth psychology become a subject, just the opposite of the earlier notion. Jung maintained that "man is at once an actor and a spectator, a participant-observer, who cannot, in the interest of truth remain a stranger to himself."[2] This conception of the ego has many facets, only one of which is the function of perception, and it is intimately bound up with functions of personality in general. In his typological system, Jung postulates "eight different but equally normal ways of experiencing and perceiving the world. There are four functional types–thinking, feeling, sensation, and intuition."[3] Thinking is a function of cognition (i.e., logic), while feeling is a function of conation (i.e., valuing). Sensation and intuition are both functions of perception. If they are outwardly directed (i.e. extroverted), they are functions for perceiving the outer world. If they are inwardly directed, (i.e., introverted), they are functions for perceiving the inner world. This boils down to the fact that there are two functions by which inner objects are perceived, introverted sensation and introverted intuition. Usually, introverted intuition, in this system, is considered to be the only function of inner perception. It is the function by which the ego is able to perceive the images representing the inner world directly, with all their possibilities for realization, and leads to a strong premonition of the probable. We may recall William Blake's aphorism concerning this function with its occasional gift of prophecy: "What is now proved was once only imagined."[4]

However, introverted sensation is also described as a function of inner perception, and I have long felt that its role should not be neglected in favor of the more obvious function of intuition. This form of sensation perceives outer objects, not as thinks in themselves, but as connected with inner reality in a special way. These objects are subjectively experienced forms to be particularized in present time, i.e., at the moment of perceiving, unlike the forms perceived by intuition that are always changing in accordance with their capacity for becoming something else, oriented to future, rather than present, time. An example of inner perception by way of sensation may be represented by Plato's idea of eternal images as embodying perfect models (*eidola*), of which all external tangible things are mere imitations. It is also suggestive of Kant's philosophical concept of the *Ding an sich,* that which is a law unto itself.

Because the imaginative nature of introverted intuition makes exorbitant demands on the credulity of average men, those who employ it exclusively as a means of perception are likely to be accused of mysticism in the sense of obscurantism. The practical importance of its activity is therefore frequently overlooked. For instance, this function in a medicine man or shaman is a practical necessity in a tribal society existing without our technological advantages. Medieval alchemy "swarmed with hypostases," which could not be substantiated in any material sense, yet it opened the way to pharmacology, chemistry, and, if we are to believe Jung, in our own day to some of the most important aspects of depth psychology.

Whoever relies exclusively upon introverted sensation, on the other hand, tries to represent the inner images in so realistic and so pure a form that they seem prosaic, and he is critized for being slow, dull, and unimaginative. He merely seems to be interested in one tangible image and to present it so repetitively that we become bored by it and impatient with him because we do not see his inner vision. There is even a kind of staleness in the reiteration of Plato's concept of the *eidola,* those unchanging ideal images we can never hope to see. Similarly the painter, Cezanne, totally failed to impress his contemporaries because he insisted on painting the same view of Mt. St. Victoire a hundred times, neglecting many marvelous other landscapes the South of France affords. Yet the message delivered by the sensation function from some inner source may be unsuspectingly powerful in its ultimate impact. Plato is still the philosopher to whom, since his time, all other philosophers have first gone to study. In those few paintings of Cezanne we can now see the whole development of modern painting in its transition from 19th century realism to 20th century abstract impressionism, and he shows why the change became necessary. In this type of perception through sensation, which seems so limited and yet, which contains so much inner meaning, we might recall another aphorism of Blake: "Eternity is in love with the productions of time."

From the study of these functions, I have concluded that one of them alone is unable to perceive the whole inner image. In people who are not over-identified with either one, both are necessary to complement each other and correct each other's extremism; together they exhibit the full spectrum emanating from the inner objects. Intuition brings into view a dazzling series of images for consideration, the stuff of fantasy in its most colorful form. Sensation selects the one image from all the others which can reduce its many possibilities into one reality. Sensation gives reality to the images which, if left to intuition, would convey the impression of psychedelic nonsense. We never perceive the true inner world face to face, but by playing one function against the other, or using first one and then the other, we may arrive at an approximation of the truth more completely than we could by relying upon one or the other alone.

In order to demonstrate the value of this double form of perception, I would have to produce a great deal of clinical material, since these functions are, by their very nature, being wholly concerned with inner things, the least accessible to objective study. I can only state that I do have sufficient evidence from my analytic practice that there are two functions which, together, do form an effective bridge to an inner world where there are, as I hope to show next, real inner objects to perceive.

The Contents of Inner Perception

At first sight, as I have indicated, we may be tempted to describe contents of the inner world solely by reference to objects of the outer world. True enough, there is a personal aspect of the unconscious that contains fragments of memory and the imprint of personal complexes associated with family patterns, and there is a considerable reflection of outer events and environmental conditions. But if we continue to examine these contents with the functions of inner perception, we find that there are certain images which do not fit into this personal frame of reference. They seem to lead a life of their own. Let us take, for instance, the appearance of the ego in dreams. The ego is one of many other alter-egos, figures derived from the dreamer's experience of interpersonal relationship. To interpret such dreams, we accordingly have to reduce these figures to certain traits, tendencies, or potentialities that are being repressed for emotional reasons, or are attempting to compensate for certain failures in development. But there are also many dreams that are really fantasies in which, instead of alter-ego figures, there is one figure usually antithetic to the dreamer and without any demonstrable connection with his personal life situation. Here the dreamer is the protagonist in a nonpersonal drama with an antagonist, which Jung has called the "Shadow." In his words it "involves an experience of a special kind, namely, the recognition of an alien 'other' in oneself, or the objective presence of another will,"[5] which leads to a confrontation that seems to have the purpose of abolishing the dissociation between the personal unconscious and the inner world of archetypal symbols. Many examples from world literature come to mind, but one will have to suffice. Mephistopheles in Goethe's Faust is an archetypal shadow-figure. The longevity of the Faust legend dating from the middle ages which, beside Marlowe's and Goethe's versions, has again been rewritten in our time by Thomas Mann in his Dr. Faustus, points to man's confrontation with a shadow-figure which can only be described as an autonomous complex of the objective psyche.

In addition to the shadow-figure, which always appears as the same sex as the dreamer, there is a contrasexual figure, the *anima,* an impersonal feminine figure in men's dreams, and the *animus,* a corresponding masculine figure in women's dreams. These images are frequently projected to real historical figures or the heroes and heroines of literature. Goethe was also well aware of this figure which holds so important a place in his writings. Every German schoolboy has to learn the names of the actual women who inspired each period of Goethe's work, but Goethe himself knew better than to identify his inspiration as coming from any one of them. He called it *das Ewig-weibliche* (*the eternal feminine*), showing his awareness of its nature as an archetypal image.

The archtypal images are the true objects of the inner world. But if we see them only as images, they present us with an intellectual problem of the first order. Being so commonly expressed in the figures of world mythology, they seem to be more the products of various culture patterns than to exist in their own right. This has led me to suggest that besides the archetypes, there is an area of inner psychic activity that really is historically, and therefore culturally, determined, producing a type of symbolism that could not have been consciously transmitted, but is nevertheless unconsciously transmitted to children from parents and educators. Freudian revisionists such as Horney, Fromm, Erikson, and the Jungian revisionist, Neumann, together with certain professors of ancient philosophy and cultural anthropologists, have contributed to the understanding of this aspect of the inner life. In some cases they also have been able to show links between these cultural determinants and personal life experiences. But there is still much to be done in demonstrating this phenomenon psychologically.

Jung, as I have said, speaks frequently of these historical images as archetypal images, but this is not what he meant by the term, archetype, and so this has often tended to obscure his real point of view. Originally, he referred to the archetypes simply as primordial images, following Burckhardt. He may also have remembered Adolf Bastian's classification of mythology as comprising two sorts of image, *constant* or *variable.* The constants he called *elementary ideas* and the variables, *ethnic ideas.* Jung's archetypal images are similar to Bastian's elementary ideas, which are nowhere to be found in a pure state but are, according to Joseph Campbell, manifested "only by way of the rich variety of their extremely interesting, frequently startling, yet always finally recognizable reflections in the panorama of human life."[6] Jung stressed the psychological, spontaneous primary nature of archetypes, which antedate and ultimately give birth to ethnic forms, and that is why he called them primordial.

There is a distinct division between this viewpoint and that of the Freudian revisionists who derive mythology exclusively from the culture pattern, and therefore, are dealing largely with ethnic, rather than elementary, ideas. For them there can be no true inner objects, since they think all mythological patterns, whether consciously or unconsciously, have been introjected into the individual psyche from without. This may not give rise to open disagreement, however, because the images, whether they are archetypal or ethnic, frequently appear to be identical. This is especially apparent in Neumann's revision of Jung, where the archetypal and ethnic ideas are freely interchanged, and so he avoids the occasional dogmatism of Jung's insistence on keeping them separate.

This may be illustrated, though too briefly, in reference to the two dream figures I have mentioned, the "shadow" and the anima. In their historically familiar forms, they convey certain well-known meanings for the cultural life of mankind. Accordingly they are not archetypes but stereotypes. But if, like masks, we remove these stereotypes, we may reveal the true archetypal image behind them. Then certain basic qualities of human psychology come into view.

The shadow, behind its demonic mask, reveals a kind of interior conscience with its concern for man's spiritual welfare, and it presents him with a fear of being damned if he does not find some form of redemption. In the Old Testament before Satan became anthropomorphized, he was a verb, sātān, "to hinder, to oppose an existing intention,"[7] and also a noun meaning "persecution by hindering free forward movement." This form of conscience is very different from Freud's super-ego, which is also conscience, but introjected from definite cultural patriarchal traditions. Conscience in the archetypal sense, is not a learned reaction, but an innate property of the psyche and therefore corresponds to a true inner content. The shadow-figure, therefore, challenges man to become conscious of this particular inner content with its basic religious quality, or, as one might put it, awakening him to the knowledge of good and evil.

The anima-figure appears in so many bewildering and seductive disguises that it might seem impossible to find any one psychological meaning for her. Goethe, who, as I have indicated, had seen more faces of Eve than most men, at the end of his great work, Faust, boldly asserts what he felt to be her essential quality when he says, "the eternal feminine draws us onward and upward."[8] This is the psychology of inspiration which implies that if he can withstand her seductions, which means his temptation to project her image on real women, or merely love himself narcissistically, she may reveal to a man his creative capacity to surpass himself, whether upon the extroverted road of enthusiasm or the introverted road of ecstasy. In terms of the psychological experience of the *anima*, these roads are identical.

Numerous other archetypal images have been described by Jungian writers in the attempt to reveal their inherent psychological quality, e.g. The Divine Child, The Primordial Maiden, The Patterns of Initiation, The Great Mother, The Archetypal Father, and so on, but a great deal of work still needs to be done. What takes so much time and energy is learning not to fall into quasi-religious, or philosophical, or esthetic explanations of the material, and to keep firmly in mind the scientific principle that these explorations must not be pushed beyond the bounds of psychological probability. Yet it is also important, of course, to be aware that unknown factors lie behind all phenomenology.

Inner perception in terms of depth psychology would not be complete without some account of the process of change we see reflected in dreams and fantasies during the course of an individual analysis. The patient, or, as we prefer to call him, the analysand, produces unconscious material that reveals many images marking stages of progression alternating with regression in a cyclic movement, leading to integration of all the factors involved. The images activated in this process cannot be simply or singly perceived; a more appropriate term for the way we observe them is not perception, but apperception. Apperception is perceiving in multiple ways, and this is what we must do with inner images, as they move and change and regroup themselves by some unexpected and frequently humorous play of contrasts. I am indebted, not to a psychologist, but to a professor of management science, C. West Churchman, for an example of apperception in this sense:

> Perception means looking at something in a purposive way. . . . Apperception happens to us all the time. We watch a cat at play. All of a sudden, it is not a cat but a dancer, creating a marvelous pattern of furry motion. We watch a mathematician earnestly struggling to solve a set of equations . . . . he's not a mathematician but an artist carefully placing strings of symbols in a marvelous mosaic. A hobo is a cheap, downgraded, dirty form of humanity; Charlie Chaplin lets us apperceive him to be subtle, sensitive, and pathetically comical.[9]

During the course of analysis, quite a few of my analysands learn to apply a similar kind of apperception to the imagery of their dreams or fantasies. Instead of trying to analyse this material intellectually, they let it speak to them; instead of directing it, they collaborate with it. The result is a creative, on-going mood of adventure which Jung has called active imagination. Personally, I do not urge people to use this as a method, but when it begins spontaneously (and it often does), I encourage them to keep it going until they have made the most of it. The only test of its validity lies with the subjective experience of the analysand, if he finds in it a new source of self-realization of the kind that conveys a sense of wholeness and unity transcending the usual state of dissociation between conscious thoughts and unconscious images.

If we apperceive the contents of the personal unconscious, the result varies from the banal to the comic, but if the contents are archetypal, a more serious and more complex type of reaction is found. I leave you to imagine how many strange mixtures of personal and archetypal imagery may also be found in this process. I have singled out one dream image, by which I hope to show the value of apperception in resolving a personal problem by insight derived from an archetypal image.

The case is that of a young man in his early thirties, who was suffering from a neurosis based on his having lived, up to this time, a provisional life. Although he had a satisfactory career and marriage, he had all kinds of resistances and escape fantasies through which he tried to avoid fully accepting them. Much had been done on the personal level to free him from this provisional attitude, and he was most cooperative, yet discouraging regressions were frequent. The following dream gripped his fantasy, and with my help a number of important apperceptions led to a much greater sense of conviction that he was now ready to be caught in a fateful encounter with his present and future life.

In the dream he had an important test to pass which meant life or death to him. He had to lodge an axe in a tree. He says:

> I began trying haphazardly to put the axe in the tree, starting at one point and going all around the tree until I finally succeeded. This all took place in an open forest. Then I and three other men were brought to a castle. One of the keepers was asked why he or she did not tell us we would be brought here, because once here there would be no return or no escape. The woman keeper said it was not for her to tell us.
>
> The inner castle was enclosed by a high circular wall. Besides the four of us captives, there were now three keepers. Together we made a group of seven. All of the people in this group were represented each by the signs for the sun, moon and planets, seven in all. We were still ordinary people, but each one of us was connected with a different planet. There would be no return from the castle. I wondered how it was that we came to this fate when we started out with such an innocent earthly beginning.

In this dream the personal problem of the dreamer is answered in a symbolic way, suggestive of a story from medieval mythology, perhaps from the Arthurian romances. The dreamer is in the guise of a quest-hero such as Gawain, who is looking for the Grail Castle. This is suggested by the initiatory trial of strength, a test of manhood and of dedication.[10] The tree is perhaps the Tree of Life, which requires that he affirm its importance for him in an act of will, which is represented by finding the right place and putting his axe into its bark. There are numerous old stories and legends in which such symbolism is found, where the novice for an initiation has to perform an act for which he has no previous experience, with a meaning similar to this dream; in one and the same act it is as if he chooses his fate and his fate chooses him.

He and his earthly comrades, four in number, comprise in the language of dream symbolism, the totality of his personality, all of himself, so to speak. Psychologically it represents the ego with its four functions. Brought into the castle, this totality is joined by three figures which in dream symbolism represent a spiritually oriented trinity. While he emphasizes that they are all human beings, male and female, the natures of the three keepers is stressed, which points to a pair of opposites that is included in this number and lends it a symbolism of the feminine, namely the *anima.* The castle with its circular wall suggests a centered, protective device for keeping all the people involved in this encounter in one psychic system. The four outsiders and the three keepers then are integrated into one group, represented by their total number, seven. Presumably this means the achievement of unity between the earthly aspect of this man's knowledge of himself, and an inner spiritual aspect about which he knows as yet nothing. But the dream tells him, or shall we say, he learns by his own interior apperception that the integration has taken place, insofar as the sun, moon, and planets, seven in all, belong together in a meaningful relationship.

You will, no doubt, have noticed that much of this symbolism must have been introjected from cultural traditions to which the dreamer has been exposed. He was aware of the Arthurian romances and he had undoubtedly read somewhere, although he could not say where, some account of the seven planets, a notion derived from classical mythology and philosophy that found its way into Christian iconography by way of astrology and alchemy. The original number symbolism of the three, the four, and the seven, can be traced even farther back in history to much more primitive sources. The peculiar symbolism of the four and the three added together, making seven, is a symbolism so abstruse that I myself would not know where to look for it in the alchemical or other texts. I can be sure in any case that this analysand did not know of it. Or if by any strange chance he had seen something to suggest it, the particular union of the four, representing his earthly self, and the three, representing his spiritual potential was original with him, an example of what we mean by archetypal symbolism, as distinct from ethnic or cultural symbolism. The whole symbolism of initiation is contained in this dream image, seven being the number associated with initiation as an inner process.

The analysand is thus brought into a place from which escape is no longer possible, meaning no escape backward regressively to his provisional boyhood pattern of behavior. Initiation in this sense means growing up with a new moral and spiritual determination to integrate the ego with the self. This is a Jungian concept which was beautifully described by John Perry in his lecture at one of the previous psychology conferences several years ago, in which he demonstrated, in a study on schizophrenia,[11] that the self in this psychology is the central archetype that has an ordering effect on all the others.

In discussing this dream with my analysand, I carefully avoided introducing these theoretical concepts and encouraged him rather to take from the dream only what possibilities for further exploration specifically spoke to his condition. I have no doubt that such a dream will have many delayed effects upon the consciousness of this young man, and it would be unfortunate if he became too bookish and tried to intellectualize his experience prematurely. He should also remain true to his own apperceptions.

It is in such ways that the functions of perception, together with the function of apperception, work in the long run to ensure an ongoing dialectic between conscious and unconscious modes of thought or behavior.

References

1. Whyte, L. L. 1960. The Unconscious Before Freud. Tavistock Publications, Ltd. London.
2. Matson, F. W. 1964. The Broken Image. : 163. Braziller. New York
3. Mann, H. & O. Siegler. 1968. J. Anal. Psychol. Tavistock Publications, Ltd. London.
4. Blake, W. 1932. The Marriage of Heaven and Hell. Proverbs of Hell. Blake's Poetry and Prose. Geoffrey Keynes, Ed. Nonesuch. London.
5. Jung, C. G. 1968. "The philosophical tree," Alchemical Studies. *In* Collected Works, : 349. Bollingen Series XX. Princeton University Press, N. J.
6. Campbell, J. 1957. The Masks of God, Primitive Mythology. Viking Press.
7. Shärf-Kluger, R. 1967. Satan in The Old Testament. Northwestern University Press. Chicago.
8. Ortega y Gasset, J. 1949. "Goethe and the modern age." *In* Concerning a Bicentennial Goethe. Regnery. Chicago.
9. Churchman, C. W. 1967. On the Ethics of Large Scale Systems, Science Spaces Laboratory. Privately Printed. University of California Press. Internal Working Paper No. 37, vol. II.
10. Henderson, J. L., M.D. 1967. Thresholds of Initiation. Wesleyan University Press. Middletown, Conn.
11. Perry, J. W., M.D. 1962. Reconstitutive Process in the Psychopathology of the Self," Annals N. Y. Acad. Sci. New York.

Discussion

Dr. Harms: I would like to point out a factor that seems important to me in regard to the recognition of the bordering of and the transition from external or sense-perception to introspective perception. I would like to refer back to and present the observation and description by Wilhelm von Helmholtz, the importance of whose psychological postulations for perception studies is the object of my contribution in this monograph. In his Handbook of Optics in which he describes his observations on the Wahrnehmmung or "visual sensation," Helmholtz points to the fact that in the way we naively observe life, we are not psychologically ready for scientific observation. One can make this point more easily understood by pointing to the so-called microscope eye adjustment. When a person first looks through a microscope, he is frequently unable to observe any of the viruses he ought to see. A certain adjustment and positioning of the eye is necessary in order to "learn" how to observe through a microscope. It is the same with our usual general scientific observation. We must train ourselves to see scientifically, so to speak. There is something going on inside our psychological nature. We are turning from the naive application of our senses to the observation of the psychological functioning of these senses, which is an observation of our own psychological nature; and second, we are changing our "seeing" to one suitable to scientific observation. This is the point at which actual introspective perception begins. This factor seems to have been of the utmost importance to Wilhelm von Helmholtz. He strongly emphasized it by giving this instruction for proper scientific observing. For us it is still more. It is the uniquely clear presentation of the point at which the transition from outer to inner introspective observation begins, the point at which we come to experience the firts actual inner-world perception.

DR. HENDERSON: Thank you, Dr. Harms. That does add something useful. As a psychotherapist and analyst, I'm not in a position to build a bridge between the psychological picture as I see it and the experimental data done in the field of sense perception. And that is, of course, a limitation of my work.

DR. TRESSELT: What kind of research work has been followed up to try to support your theories and beliefs?

DR. HENDERSON: There is some work being done by a number of different psychologists in an attempt to verify the psychological types and functions. There is a recent publication by a psychologist named Harriet Mann and two other workers at Princeton, who were not Jungians but experimental psychologists. They did a very nice study on the types and functions called The Many Worlds of Time. Also, in California, Dr. Wayne Detloff is apparently doing a more filtered kind of work, gathering a great deal of data from a great many different patients, including State Hospital patients and criminal cases and trying to get more external proof of these theories.

PERCEIVING AND THINKING: THEIR INTERRELATIONSHIP AND ORGANISMIC ORGANIZATION*

Walter S. Boernstein, M.D.
Research Center for Mental Health
New York University, New York, N. Y.

"The problems which would be raised here are old enough; there is no immediate danger of their solution."[1]

INTRODUCTION: COMBINATION OF HUMAN PSYCHOLOGY, COMPARATIVE PHYSIOLOGY, AND PHYLOGENETICS

When man began thinking about his position in, and his relationship to, the world outside, when, in other words, mythical ideation was gradually replaced by discursive thinking, he started to wonder: What is real in the world that surrounds us? What makes the world tick? The distinction between *perceiving*, and *thinking*, which Parmenides, about 500 B.C., introduced into philosophy, gave rise to a further question which has haunted philosophical minds for nearly 2,500 years: Do we learn about the world as it *really* is by perceiving or by thinking? How are the two faculties related to each other? If the messages conveyed by perception and the results of our thinking contradict each other, which shall we trust? For it was taken for granted that each of these faculties is a static entity, clearly set off from one another, and from other functions of the organism, and that each faculty is homogeneous, so that what is found to be characteristic of one sense would be valid for all senses. Nor has it ever been doubted that whatever we perceive is spatially given. It is the optic sense that, as a rule, serves as a paradigm for all senses. (". . . all our sense perceptions are in the same boat, and must be treated on the same principle . . .")[2] It is "perception" that conveys to us knowledge of the physical world in which we live.[3] "Perception" is "always concerned" with *information,* says the philosopher D. W. Hamlyn.[4] Other authors claim the same for thinking. But is "knowledge," or is "information," the criterion for perceiving, for thinking? Information on, knowledge of, what? The ambiguity of the term "knowledge" and how many degrees it implies have been impressively demonstrated by A. J. Ayer.[5]

The present paper tries to show that a purely intellectualistic approach to the interrelationship between perceiving and thinking does not do justice to the problem. This paper is based on three facts:

1. Perceiving and thinking are functions of the organism in question. This means that they themselves are somatopsychological in nature, i.e., they must be studied from both psychological and somatic angles. And as organismic functions they are correlated with other organismic functions, consequently correlated with pertinent anatomical structures. In other words, neither perceiving nor thinking is an isolated activity.

2. The faculties of both perceiving and thinking are arranged in a hierarchical order, which extends from preperceptual and prethought–primitive, purely so-

* The present abbreviated paper is based on my idea of the principle of "specific sensorimotor sense synergies," which was the starting point of my very first scientific endeavor, viz., to provide proof that the cortical taste center in man cannot be located in the rhinencephalon but must be located in the parietal lobe, near the areas for mastication and tongue movements. The monograph, presenting facts of comparative physiology, and experiments on 13 patients with pertinent brain lesions, was unfortunately lost before completion. Due to unfavorable external conditions, the publication of the present paper in its full and elaborated form, including the complete bibliography, has also been prevented.

matic–processes to the most highly differentiated mental functions. The transition from the low to the high processes can be demonstrated within the single individual as well as in the course of evolution.

3. This hierarchical order is determined by the development of organs and pertinent functions during phylogenesis. This proceeds in various ways: (a) by encephalization, with internalization (psychologization) of functions; and (b) by the more or less close fusion of primitive functions with highly differentiated ones.

Example (*a*): In the dark-adapted frog, contraction of the myoids of the cones in the retina, as in "light-adaptation," is also elicited by increase of the body tonus, such as violent struggling of the frog chained on its board, or by injection of strychnine or adrenaline, whereas the injection of the muscle-paralyzing curare would have no effect (Observation by Th. Engelmann in 1885). I ventured the hypothesis that what is a purely somatic process in the frog would in man be internalized, i.e., be a psychological phenomenon, experienced as optic imagery. The experiments to be presented below confirm this hypothesis.

Example (*b*): Even the highest mental functions of man–his faculty for perceiving high Gestalten, and his faculty for creating new ideas in science and art–are not exclusively the product of differentiation and encephalization, but of the integration of primitive somatic functions with these highly differentiated functions. This fusion of low with high functions–specialization with nonspecialization –is typical of man, and it is more realized in man's highest sense (vision) than in any of his other senses. An example of the persistence of primitive mechanisms throughout all of evolution is the reactivity of all creatures living under the sun to bright and dark stimuli. The influence of optic light on the innersecretory state of vertebrates, from frog to man, was demonstrated by this writer through the injection of the "light-blood" of man, rabbit, and frog into the eye-bulbs of "dark-frogs.[6]

Erich von Hornbostel[7] pointed out that nonoptic sensory stimuli are also perceived by man as "bright" and "dark," respectively. This paper tries to show that the brightness quality has its physiological equivalent in its tonus-increasing effect, the darkness quality in its tonus-decreasing effect; and that tonus-increasing factors, even if they are not sensory in nature, are distinguished by their brightness quality, and vice versa.[8] According to Hornbostel, these are "basic sensory functions," belonging to the "most ancient aspects of physiological processes." I called them "a-modal."[8] This paper is largely based on the correlation between bright-dark stimuli and body tonus.

Internalization through encephalization and persistence of ancient functions are two of the roots from which the faculty of thinking has developed: Phylogenetic facts help us to understand the mechanism of thinking.

The necessity for the synthesis of *phylogenetics* and *human psychology* is a postulate, dating back some 100 years, to Wilhelm Wundt (quoted from K. Lorenz[9]). But his remained a lonely voice in the wilderness until, some decades ago, Julian Huxley proclaimed that ". . . without some knowledge of evolution one cannot hope to arrive at a true picture of human destiny . . ." During the last 30 years, Konrad Lorenz[9] has most emphatically stressed the fact that the complex laws that control man's mental life, including his social behavior, are the same as those that control the life of all organisms.

This paper represents one of the first attempts, I believe, to approach the interrelationship between "perceiving" and "thinking" from three biological aspects: human psychology, comparative physiology, and phylogenetics.

Questions Regarding the Interrelationship Between Perceiving and Thinking

A large number of questions arises as a consequence of this three-fold approach. Only a few can be raised here: Are perceiving and thinking two different faculties? Or are they controlled by the same principle? Has thinking developed from perceiving? Or is perceiving itself a thought process? Can we perceive without thinking, think without processes in the sense organs? Are there levels of perceiving, of thinking? If so, what criterion would distinguish them? Is all perceiving "spatial"? What is imagery? Is it characteristic of all sensory fields? What is its relation to (extero-) perception, and to thinking? Is, for instance, dream imagery, in which problems can be solved, a kind of thinking? How can imagery be educed? What is the effect of inadequate stimuli on a given sensory system? How are perceiving, thinking and feeling related to one another? What role does the environment play in the evolution of perceiving, of thinking? This is only a small selection of questions concerned with the interrelationship between perceiving and thinking and the organism as a whole.

The Role of Structure in Perceiving and Thinking: "High" and "Low" Senses

In early papers (literature in Boernstein[8]) I proclaimed that the perceiving of "high Gestalten," i.e., of highly differentiated dynamic structures in space, or "quasi-space" (audition) is not a purely sensory function, but can be achieved only by the "high" or "spatial" senses; i.e., by those senses in which the sensory component is firmly integrated into one functional unit with its pertinent tonic component on the same level of differentiation. "Gestalt perception is an act." Cognition of objects would therefore not be possible without a pertinent functional involvement of the body tonus. I proposed the term "specific sensoritonic sense synergies," underlying those perceptual processes. (Years later, Heinz Werner and Jean Piaget applied the term "sensu-tonus" to all sensory systems although without differentiation.)

It is the motor (tonic) component that enables us to "comprehend" disparate but allied objects and events into one dynamic structure. The optic system is more widely and more intensely correlated with the body tonus than is any other sensory system. The optic sense is, consequently, the highest sense of man—the "spatial sense" *par excellence*. The *"low senses,"* on the other hand, olfaction, taste, the temperature senses, and so on, convey no more than weak, if any, spatial-dynamic structures, i.e., "pre-," if not "a-spatial" percepts. The "low percepts" are little or not at all structured or contoured; consequently, they can not be transposed.

Conclusion: Instead of asking how are "perceiving" and "thinking" interrelated, the question should be, *what type,* or level of perceiving is involved with that of thinking? The optic sense particularly conveys a "syn-opsis," that is, the perceiving "at one glance" of a dynamic structure, both in (extero-)perception and in imagery. Spatial senses, and particularly the optic sense, enable the person to perceive transposable "invariants," the precondition for perceptual cognition, and for discursive thinking.† The importance of the correlation between tonus

† The importance of the "structure" concept for a psychoanalytic theory has recently been discussed by Robert R. Holt.[10] Benjamin B. Rubinstein[11] predicts that "one day the gap between psychoanalytic theory and neurophysiology will be bridged." Perhaps the tonus-concept as presented here might help to bridge the gap; see below on induced optic images.

apparatus and spatial senses, particularly vision of human beings, has impressively been confirmed by phylogenetic facts.

The Influence of the Environment on the Phylogenesis of Thinking, Determined by the Phylogenesis of Space Orientation

The decisive role of the sense of vision in the evolution of thinking was demonstrated by the classical studies of Konrad Lorenz in 1950 (quoted from Lorenz[9]). That spatial orientation and, subsequently, thinking have evolved in phylogenesis, Lorenz has shown on the basis of the opticomotor integration that develops under the influence of the spatial structurization of the environment. Where spatial obstacles have to be overcome, the animal evolves the faculty of space orientation. Animals living in the free ocean or on open plains, moving at random in any direction, do not evolve movements adapted to the outer world; they have no problems to solve in catching prey. From teleostean fish to primates, the capability to overcome an obstacle on the way to reaching a goal stands, conditions being otherwise equal, in direct proportion to the complexity of the spatial structurization in the environment. What originally, in fish, is a combination of reflexes ("taxis") becomes an intended movement in the course of phylogenesis; and, finally, in primates, including man, an internalized movement; i.e., a movement is first anticipated, and then carried out. In other words, the "central representation of space"[9] makes the internalization of a spatial problem and its solution possible. Shall we speak, then, of "opticomotor imagining," or of "deliberating" the solution? This process of anticipating the solution "in the 'imagined' space" ["*im 'vorgestellten' Raum*"] before acting is the beginning of thinking. The same phenomenon remains "the indispensable basis even for our most complex thought processes."[9] Space orientation, based on the spatial senses and the motorium, is, in other words, the root from which the faculty of thinking evolves.

The Optic System as the Receiver of Nonoptic A-Modal Stimuli

In Animals

In the Introduction, it was mentioned that light adaptation in the frog retina can be elicited by tonus increase; i.e., that tonus increase acts on that retina like optic light. I supposed that the melanophores in the amphibian skin are controlled by the same principle. My experiments showed indeed that the bright odor 1-citronellol has a light effect, and the dark odor scatol, a dark effect on the skin melanophores of African clawed toads. The corresponding result was obtained by P. von Schiller's[12] psychological experiments on fishes (10 minnows).‡

In Man

The experiments reveal that such nonoptic stimuli that in animals increase the body tonus, also increase it in man, and are perceived as "bright," and vice versa. Furthermore, the same stimuli can evoke in man bright, pleasant optic images, and vice versa for dark, tonus-decreasing stimuli.

The following experiments on "induced optic imagery" confirm these statements.

Method: The subjects lay relaxed, in complete darkness until the "entoptic

‡ A more detailed report on these and other experiments is presented in Boernstein.[8]

phenomena" ("phosphenes") were reduced to dim stars or clouds or to homogeneous grey, without movement: "Dark adaptation." To attain this takes, on the average, a maximum of 45–60 minutes. Then a bright odor (rose oil or citronellol-1) or a bright taste (a lump of sugar) is offered; or a dark odor (scatol) or dark taste (magn. sulf.); or other bright or dark stimuli (such as tensing the arm against resistance, or pertinent sounds). The optic images would appear after a latency time of a few seconds to two minutes.

Protocols: 1. (*Citronellol*): "I see very clearly a pastel red, very distinct, like a fluorescent light . . . A perfect picture, like a painting, as if my eyes were open!"

2. (*Rose Oil*): "Things get slowly whiter and snowy. I see a white rabbit with black eyes and long ears. A snowy mountain in the background." (The foreground is partly drawn as a homogeneous dark.)

3. (*First Rose Oil, then Scatol*): (*Rose Oil*): "I see a bottle of 'Old Spice'; very white, milky white; the writing is blue . . ." (Image appears after two minutes); (*Scatol*): "Just now I see a black and white flashing, white in black. Black clouds in a sunset; the sun is red, going down. . . ."

4. This experiment demonstrates the close correlation between brightness and pertinent emotion, and vice versa with darkness. Rose oil and scatol are given alternatively. (*Rose Oil*): "The smell reminds me of flowers; I see flowers, yellow and white–I see a mountain with pine trees; very pleasant;–I see a light flashing–I see all white." (*Scatol*): "It is dark now. It looks like nighttime. I see buildings; they are in deep shadow." (*Rose Oil*): "It is light again. The buildings look lit up. It is daytime; pleasant;–all white– I see a church from inside; stained-glass window in various colors." (*Scatol*): "The church gets dark. People are running out of it. It is unpleasant. It looks like danger. . . ."

Conclusion: These experiments demonstrate that bright optic images, and corresponding emotions, also "bright," can be elicited by nonspecific, tonus-increasing stimuli (sensory and nonsensory in nature); "dark" stimuli have the opposite effect on imagery and emotion: The psychological state is expressed in the optic image. The results were always positive in the "eidetics" of Jaensch's terminology.[13] They were sometimes positive in altogether 70 out of 100 subjects, with the effects depending on the stimulus agent, which would act differently on different subjects.

The induced optic images, furthermore, run the whole gamut from fragmented, still phosphenes to vivid, well-structured complex scenes, even in motion, just as we find it in dream imagery. In the induced optic images it also was sometimes possible to bring repressed conflict situations, tinged with strong affects, to the fore ("sugar experiment," Boernstein[8]).

The fact that 30 out of 100 subjects were completely "refractory" fits in with Jaensch's findings of the "disintegrated type" of people (in contrast to the "integrated" or "opticomotor" type) in whom not only the optic system fails to play the predominant role in perception, but also the entire somato-psychic set-up of the person significantly differs from those of the integrated type. The basic difference in the personality type significantly shows in the writings and other productions of creative people.

The Split in Philosophy: Empiricism and Rationalism

The entire history of philosophy can be considered as one single dispute between empiricism and rationalism (or "idealism").[14,15]

Empiricists. Only by perceiving the concrete, momentarily given objects, and by abstracting from them would we arrive, with probability of sorts, at general laws (The method of "induction.") Our "cause-effect" concept would be the result of associations (David Hume), brought about by objects that always follow one another in the same sequence. Thinking would begin ". . . as specific sensory input from one or more of the classical receptors (eye, ear, etc.);" and perceiving, learning, thinking, and emotion are isolated factors.[16] Cognition would be involved in all those processes by which the sensory input is "transformed . . . stored . . . and used," and all psychological phenomena would be "cognitive."[17] According to the empiricists, our ideas would, thus, be connected by "associations," would originate from "impressions" from the world outside. The role of emotions is ignored, and quantification would be the goal and criterion of science. Concepts such as "value," "biological meaning," and, last but not least, "structure" have no place in empiricism. This way of thinking has led to Ivan Pavlov's *Reflexology*, and to *Behaviorism* that plays such a dominant role in this country. It is of the scientists of this type that Walter B. Cannon[18] remarks: They are "accumulators"; they "sit down and think . . . what the next move shall be." Their creativity lies, I submit, in their capability to abstract from the objectively given material they have gathered.

Rationalists. Percepts are deceptive, the rationalists insist. Only through thinking would we arrive at the insight into the essential, the invariant, the "idea" (Plato) behind the perceptible, ever-changing objects, and thus to the principle controlling the world. This insight into a general principle could be applied to individual observations (The method of "deduction.") However, logical thinking alone does not lead to the discovery of a general principle, as Albert Einstein has emphasized. What is needed in addition is "intuition." The creative rationalists would, then, be those thinkers who arrive at their insight through intuition. The present discussion deals with the creative intuitionalists among the rationalists. An outstanding representative of this type of thinking is the physiologist Claude Bernard.[19] The experimental method in medicine, he sees based on "the tripod of 'feeling' . . . reason and experience;" i.e., on the fusion of emotion, thinking, perceiving. But "feeling . . . always holds the initiative and engenders 'the *a priori* idea (i.e., hypothesis) or intuition' ". This type of thinking is referred to by other authors also as "idealistic."

Conclusion: The two ways of philosophical creative thinking, empiricism and intuitionalistic rationalism, proceed in two opposite directions: The empiricists, to whom only the perceptible is real and for whom our mind is originally an "empty table" (*tabula rasa*–Locke), teach that the psychological phenomena originate on the periphery, that the impulses travel centripetally. The rationalists, on the contrary, claim that an endogenous process, thinking, is the source of cognizing the world, that the world is met by centrifugal impulses.

The Incompatability Between Representatives of the Two Types of Thinking

That the antagonism between these two types of thinking in fact encompasses differences in the entire somatopsychological make-up was seen as long ago as 1907 by William James.[20] He sees the empiricist as "tough-minded, materialistic, irreligious, skeptical . . . ," who values "facts in all their crude variety." The rationalist is characterized as "tender-minded, intellectualistic, idealistic, optimistic, religious . . . dogmatic;" he would value "abstract and eternal principles."

As sweeping as this statement seems to be, a brief glance at the history of philosophy supports it.

Intuitionalists. Pythagoras (530 B.C.), starting from his observation of the vibration of chords in musical instruments, deduces from it his principle of "number" controlling the universe. He preaches the perfect harmony of all beings; beauty is to him "a fundamental character of reality."[21] His school is dedicated to both religion and science. The discrepancy in feeling and thinking between intuitionalist and empiricist is vividly demonstrated by the relationship between Johannes Kepler[22] and Tycho de Brahe. The intuitionalist Kepler is depicted by Albert Einstein as a finely sensitive person, passionately dedicated to the search for a deeper insight into the essence of natural events. Kepler's biographer, Carola Baumgardt, refers to him as "something of a fact and one of the most lovable . . . personalities of modern history." Tycho published his material under the sober title "Astronomies." Kepler's work bears the title "Cosmic Harmonies." This is one of the most famous examples of the complementary cooperation between theory and experience.

Another typical intuitionalist, the poet-scientist Johann Wolfgang von Goethe, would emphasize "harmony" as the guiding principle in Nature.[23a,b] His *Farbenlehre* ("Color-Theory") was so emotion-laden, in fact like a religious dogma, that it meant more to him than all his famous poetic work, and he raved against Newton.[24]

Empiricists. Little can be said about their emotional attitude toward their scientific work; they are, to repeat, more involved in facts than in emotions. However, David Hume wished "the entire Natural Philosophy" to be thrown into the fire.[25] Charles Sherrington mocked Goethe's "imaginal archetypal flowering plants . . ." as illusory. Pavlov felt repugnance against Wertheimer's Gestalt theory, just as the early Gestalt theorists felt contempt for "machine-thinking."

These few examples demonstrate that the antagonism between representatives of the two chief types of creative thinkers has not changed since the times of ancient Greece, and that it encompasses the whole personality and not just the scientific attitude.

Thus, there is a direct link between intuitionalists such as Pythagoras, Parmenides and Plato and present-day philosophers, in addition to such physicists as James C. Maxwell, Max Planck and Albert Einstein; to mathematician Henri Poincaré; to physiologists Claude Bernard and Walter B. Cannon; to psychologist Max Wertheimer; and to nonscientists, such as certain mystics and painters. These examples can easily be multiplied.

Common to the intuitionalists is that they experience dynamic structures. The intuitionalist is as a whole involved in his work, and sees the world as an emotion-laden whole, in harmony and beauty.

This fact might explain that artistic gifts are so frequent among the intuitionalists: Pythagoras played musical instruments; Claude Bernard started life writing vaudevilles; Goethe was a poet; Maxwell wrote poems; Einstein and Wertheimer were musicians; and so forth. But more indicative is what such an outstanding scientist as Max Planck[26] states: ". . . the pioneer of science needs a lively synopsis (*Anschauung*), for new ideas do not come from calculated reasoning, but from the artistically creating phantasy . . ." (translation). Cannon speaks of "a leap of the imagination, for it reaches forth into the range of possibilities. . . ." Indeed, intuitionalistic creative thinking is risky, is unorthodox.

The "leap" is fired by a strong emotion: "Emotion moves us . . ." (Charles Sherrington). Emotion and motion, correlated with each other, are two factors fundamental to intuitionalistic thinking. The third factor is optic imagination, i.e., vision. The somatic difference between his terms "visionalists" and "nonvisionalists" has been demonstrated on the E.E.G. by Grey Walter. This latter factor, the guidance of thinking by vision, is illustrated by Kepler's remarks: Working on his emotion-laden problems, he *saw* "the first dawn . . . the bright day," and eventually, "the full sun of a most wonderful vision." Similarly, Wertheimer[27] "envisages structures," "sees" a problem become "transparent," etc. What is "perceptible" here, and what is "abstract"? There is no line between the two, at least not in intuitionalistic creativity.

The fluctuating borderline among seeing, feeling, and thinking is graphically expressed in the Indo-European languages where the root "vid" gives rise to "eidetic" and "vision" (in both meanings) as well as to "idea," "idol," "ideation," and so forth.[28]

The discrepancy between "empiricistic" and "intuitionalistic" *painters* can be demonstrated by comparison, e.g. of the pointillist G. Seurat with the "visionary" William Blake.§

It goes without saying that a full exploration of the problems discussed in this paper can be obtained only by an approach from many different disciplines: psychology, physiology, endocrinology, and zoology.

Conclusion and Summary

This paper is based on the principle of the "specific sensoritonic synergies," which states that the sensory component of each sensory system is more or less closely correlated (depending on the given sense) with a tonic component on the same level of differentiation, and, through it, with the body tonus as a whole.

Experiments reported here show that this principle controls activities ranging from those in the melanophores in amphibian skin to man's most complex thought processes.

The sensori-tonic correlation is particularly close in the optic system of animals and man. Here, changes in the sensory component affect the body tonus, while changes in the body tonus affect, in turn, the state in the optic system.

In human beings of the "opticomotor" or "intuitionalistic" type these nonoptic (nonspecific, "a-modal") stimuli that increase the body tonus also educe corresponding optic imagery, and vice versa.

The "high" or "spatial" senses are distinguished from the "low" or "pre-" (or "a-") spatial senses.

Space orientation, based on the spatial senses and the body tonus (motorium), is the root from which the faculty of thinking evolves.

Two somatopsychological types of man are distinguished. The difference between these two types is manifest in thinking as well as in the degree of integration of perceiving (particularly vision), feeling, and thinking.

Acknowledgment

I feel warmly grateful and indebted to Professor Leo Goldberger without whose help the publication of the present paper would not have been possible.

References

1. Adrian, E. D. 1947. The Physical Background of Perception. Oxford Clarendon Press.
2. Whitehead, A. N., quoted from Walshe, F. 1960. Some considerations upon perception. Perspective Biol. Med. **III**: 3.
3. Brain, R. 1959. The Nature of Experience. Oxford Univ. Press. London, New York, Toronto.

§ Discussion of this fact and of the difference between creative and noncreative thinking must be omitted here.

4. Hamlyn, D. W. 1957. The Psychology of Perception. The Humanities Press, Inc. New York.
5. Ayer, A. J. 1962. The Foundations of Empirical Knowledge. McMillan and Co. Ltd. London.
6. Boernstein, W. S. 1939. Liberation by light of a melanophore-stimulating substance in the blood of mammals. (Abstr.) Proc. Am. Physiol. Soc. **126:** 437.
7. von Hornbostel, E. M. 1931. Uber Geruchshelligkeit. Pflüger's Arch. Ges. Physiol. 227.
8. Boernstein, W. S. 1967. Optic perception and optic imageries in man. Their roots and relations studied from the viewpoint of biology. Internat. J. Neurol. **VI**, 2.
9. Lorenz, K. 1965. Uber Tierisches und Menschliches Verhaltem. Ges. Abhdlgen. II. R. Piper and Co. München.
10. Holt, R. R. 1967. The development of the primary process: A structural view. Psychological Issues **V:** 2-3.
11. Rubinstein, B. B. 1967. Explanation and mere description. A metascientific examination of certain aspects of the psychoanalytic theory of motivation. Psychological Issues **V:** 2–3.
12. von Schiller, P. 1933. Intersensorielle Transposition bei Fischen. Z. vgl. Physiol. 19.
13. Jaensch, E. R. 1931. Uber die Grundlagen der Menschlichen Erkenntnis. J. A. Barth. Leipzig.
14. Heinemann, F. 1959. Erkenntnistheorie. *In* Die Philosophie im 20. Jahrhundert. Ernst Klett Verlag. Stuttgart.
15. Delius, H. 1958. Positiismus und Neopositiismus. *In* Philosophie. Fischer Bücherei. Frankfurt am Main.
16. Halstead, W. C. 1958. Some biopsychology of thinking, imagery and memory. Perspective Biol. Med. **I:** 3.
17. Neisser, U. 1966. Cognitive Psychology. Appleton-Century-Crofts. New York.
18. Cannon, W. B. 1945. The Way of an Investigator. W. W. Norton and Co. Inc. New York.
19. Bernard, C., quoted from Bunge, M. 1962. Intuition and Science. Prentice Hall, Inc. Englewood Cliffs, N. J.
20. James, W. 1907. The Dilemma in Philosophy.
21. Cassirer, E. 1944. An Essay on Man. Doubleday and Co., Inc. Garden City, N. Y.
22. Kepler, J. 1951. Carola Baumgardt, Ed.
23a. Goethe, J. W. 1869. Sämtl. Werke. J. G. Cotta. Stuttgart.
23b. Goethe, J. W. 1955. Über die Natur. Insel Verlag.
24. Friedenthal, R. 1964. Goethe–sein Leben und seine Zeit. R. Piper and Co. München.
25. Feyerabend, P. K. 1958. Naturphilosophie. *In* Philosophie. Fischer Bücherei. Frankfurt am Main.
26. Planck, M. 1949. Sinn und Grenzen der exakten Wissenschaft. Hirzel. Stuttgart.
27. Wertheimer, M. 1959. Productive Thinking. Harper & Row, Inc. New York.
28. Diemer, A. 1958. Metaphysik. *In* Philosophie. Fischer Bücherei. Frankfurt am Main.

DISCUSSION

Dr. Vernon: The entire world to any one individual is divided into two parts, that part which is inside the skin and that which is outside the skin. The problem each individual has in life is to try, with his guidance mechanism and his mind, and make a proper adjustment between the part that's inside the skin and the part that's outside to establish a good satisfying relation between the self and the non-self. However, as we heard what we heard today, it seemed that perception has more to do with the sensory impression of vision, of optical sensation, than of any other sensations that exist. And I wonder what some of us would have to say of the kind of stream of consciousness that Helen Keller might have had since she was deprived of vision and hearing.

Now as I examine my own objective in the world in the events of today, I find that some of them are pleasurable and some the opposite because I've heard the word gestalt. One of the reasons I came here from quite a distant place and took a day off from work is because I wanted to find out what "Gestalt" meant. And at the end of the day I shall make a plea that that word disappear from this type of discussion completely, because I think, historically, that it has served its purpose. I did take the trouble to find out some of the things that had been written about it, and I feel today that perhaps it served a purpose historically when certain rebels were sick and tired of hearing what some psychologists were saying. They were trying to be very scientific and measure one factor of the total human reactivity alone. And they tried to use the term gestalt to mean not a segregated image, or a segregated entity, but a constellation of sense impressions. They tried to indicate that when a human being sees things about him, he just doesn't see one thing, he sees a great many things and integrates them completely, makes a judgment, adds it to the process of thinking, and then reacts. Now, of course, I think that the thinking organ is not just the brain, the thinking organ is the entire body, the brain extends right out to the fingertips, right out to the toe tips. What does a bird think with? What does a bird react with? He reacts with every part of his body at once. But I think if we are going to be scientific, we have to do things that are measurable. I think it is a little fraudulent to take something that has to do with the qualities of the human being that are mental, reduce them to a mathematical formula, and then throw some kind of a mathematical formula on the board and say that this proves we are being scientific. I think that is fraudulent and that's one of the reasons I'd like to see "Gestalt" disappear.

The whole purpose of this scientific investigation is to improve the quality of life and to help solve social problems.

DR. BOERNSTEIN: I certainly am very grateful for any criticism, and what Doctor Vernon said about Helen Keller is correct. Maybe I did not emphasize that I meant "spatial senses," which include, of course, the so-called tactile sense, including the propreoceptive functions, which, by the way, play a great role, aside from the optic sense, in Albert Einstein's thinking.

And it plays certainly a very great role in Helen Keller's case. I use the term "dynamic structure," which is the same as "Gestalt." Since we have not only the sensory component in a sensory system, but also the motor component, we are able to see things together in one spatial structure, and to me it makes no difference whether you would call it gestalt, or dynamic structure, but without it it is impossible for a human being to live.

As far as a thing not being confined only to the brain, I certainly would not doubt it. I think that I tried to make it clear that body tonus is, at least, partly outside of the brain and I did not go into the cerebral questions. I would say that the hypothalamus and particularly its posterior portion plays a tremendous role in synopsis and in regulation also of the tonus. It is not possible to see what process is located in the brain, we think. But one cannot say we think with our entire body, one can say only that those parts of our body are particularly involved. And that certainly includes the cerebral cortex.

THE SELF, REALITY, AND PERCEPTION

Leo A. Spiegel, M.D.

Albert Einstein Medical School and Montefiore Hospital and Medical Center
Bronx, N. Y.

As usually understood, perception implies a self and an object—a self that perceives an object. The structure of an ordinary sentence, of subject, verb and predicate, reflects this daily life activity called perception.

I use "self" as an existent reality which is mental in nature. Although the self cannot be apprehended by any of the senses, still it exists and is real. Most of the time I use the term in this sense and rarely, if at all, that of conception of the self, or representation of the self.

At times I speak of the "idea of the object" becoming absorbed by the self. It is, of course, obvious that the object (say, a book) cannot be taken into the self and yet at the same time exist in the outer world. Only some aspect of my experience of the object can be so taken into myself and made part of it. On the other hand, it must be admitted that "idea of the object" is somewhat redundant, for, clearly, only ideas, feelings, and sensations connected with the object can become part of the self.

Let us consider first how self can be taken. If we eliminate all objects, what is left over in the universe is self. Going on to consider objects, it can be said similarly that when self is eliminated, what is surplus is object or objects.

Such a view, while free from error, is not satisfying. It is as if one were to define an "x" by a "y". This view actually consists in defining one undefined unknown by another undefined unknown. But, as will be seen, this kind of definition is unavoidable.

Since the self is originally made up of feelings and sensations emanating from the body, it might be thought that the existence of the self can be rescued from its dependence on the object's existence by filling it with these very feelings and sensations. But if these elements are to make up *my* self, then they cannot come from just *any* body, they must come from *my* body. And for *my* body to exist as *my* body, it must have the "my" engraved on it by *me,* by an already existing self.

No way out of this dilemma appears except to return to the reciprocal definition of self and object stated earlier, and to acknowledge that these entities must remain forever bound to each other. Self and object are necessarily complementary; neither is viable without the other.

My view of the mutual interdependence of self and object is not compatible with the usual view of early life. The usual view states: in the beginning there is a self which gradually perceives the outer world as not-self. But, I would rather put early mental life in the following way: in the beginning there is a mind which, due to its make-up, eventually develops both self and object simultaneously. Neither can exist without the other; a self without an object is inconceivable. And if I were asked what I thought about a regressed objectless state, my answer would be that no self could exist then either. What is more likely is an amorphous state of feeling in which neither self nor object is as yet differentiated. For me, primary narcissism describes an organism in which self and object have not as yet been created by the mind.

How is this early mental life without self and object to be further visualized? It is made up of a *succession* of unconnected feelings of pleasure and pain, for connected states necessarily imply self and object. Consider an infant who is stuck by a diaper pin. A feeling of pain is registered. This feeling is not connected to the object, the pin (an object for us, but not for the infant). When the pin sticks the infant again, the immediate feeling of pain *remains unconnected* to the previous feeling of pain. The synthesis of the pin and the pain and that of the first pain with the second would constitute the emergence of object and self.

The organization of a differentiated universe of self and object (self and world of animate and inanimate objects) out of an originally undifferentiated, global universe of feelings and sensations appears to come about by the working of two factors. One comes from the side of what is later to be known as the self, and the other comes from the side of what is later to be known as the object. Feelings of pleasure and pain become organized into a self. That which can be withdrawn from (in order to avoid pain) becomes organized into object.[2]

It does not seem possible to answer satisfactorily the question *why* this connectedness of feelings of pleasure and pain comes about, nor why the connectedness of repeated withdrawals from painful objects occurs. An abstract word, maturation, is merely convenient shorthand for this process of organization. *How* this maturation (rather than why) appears, has often been described as due to facilitation of associative pathways – a topic beyond the scope of this paper.

We are used to the idea of many objects, but not of many selves. For unreflecting, practical common sense, there is only one self, the "I" of daily life. Yet, there are many selves. There are, for example, a legal self, a dreaming self (for which we do not feel responsible), a waking self (for which we do), and so forth. In this paper, I will work with two other selves, a perceptual self and a cognitive self.

The fundamental difference between the two selves, the perceptual and the cognitive, can be expressed in the following way. The perceptual self perceives the object *or* the self, never both simultaneously. The cognitive self embraces *both* the object and the self simultaneously. This higher self, while recognizing the separate existence of the object, also feels the object to be part of itself. (Oral incorporative elements are at work here.) The addition of this content (the idea of the object) results in expansion of this self or, conversely in contraction of it. In the former state the idea of the object will be retained in the self, and in the latter it will tend to be extruded.

Tolstoy's life offers a good example of the latter situation. His diaries show his self to be threatened by his love for his wife; he refers to his fear of losing his self through loving her. His struggle to maintain his self *despite* his love for his wife dominated his life, and his struggle ended only when, before his death, he fled from her. Psychoanalysis has uncovered at least one important factor in determining whether incorporation of the object into the self leads to expansion or contraction of the self – the libidinal and aggressive investment of the object.

I rarely refer to perceptual and cognitive processes, but, rather, to perceptual and cognitive *selves* in this paper. My concern is with more than process. It is with the psychological nature of two fundamental aspects of experience: reality and identity. Experience belongs not to a process, but to a self. But experience varies according to whether the self is merely perceiving or is also cognizing. Thus, I visualize a self which is organized around either perception or cognition. Were I to concern myself with the processes in themselves, I would refer to them as aspects of the ego's functioning. I would not refer to them as aspects of the self's experience.

I recognize the need on certain occasions to abstract these two processes from the flow of experience, but here I am concerned with the self's experience of itself and of objects as affected by perception and cognition.

Of course, neither process exists without the other. Could one perform an imaginary experiment and separate the perceptual self from the cognitive self, one would be met with two different qualities of life experience. Identity of self and objects in time and space would not exist for a perceptual self. Consciousness of self or experiencing of object would be limited to the momentary perception of each. That each perception would be conditioned by memories is granted. However this consideration does not affect the pure immediacy of each perception and the consequent discontinuous nature of the perceptual self's experience. It is only the cognitive self which can maintain continuity and identity of self and objects, and it achieves this continuity and identity by embracing the immediate self and the object. And, as will be developed later, it is only through the creation of such identities that the universe becomes real to one.

Normally, the perceptual self functions within a universe (a framework) established by the cognitive self. When this higher self is receded from and the perceptual self becomes dominant in an adult, disturbances of the world and self appear (derealization, depersonalization), either as transient symptoms or as the initial phase of schizophrenia. These formulations will become clearer with the discussion of perception.

For the third variable perception, in the linkage of self, perception, and object, I will use a simple example: "I perceive Mary over there." As a result of this perception, I can go to her, talk to her, and so on. Thus, perception achieves, first of all, a special form of *knowledge* of the world which helps me to act intelligently within it. It is an immediate knowledge (based on the sense organs), and limited to the present. Through perception *alone,* I cannot know that Mary was there yesterday or will be there tomorrow. Through perception alone, I know nothing of Mary as a persisting identity in time and space. Such wider knowledge comes to me only through cognition. Although yielding only present knowledge, perception is influenced by memories of the past and by automatic inferential processes. Helmholtz has pointed to the latter, and Proust's description of the "*petite madeleine*" is an example of the former.

So far, only external perception has been discussed. To go on now to internal perception, let us take as an example, "I love Mary." As an expression of feeling, it is the outcome of a perception of the inner world. So perception must be redefined as giving knowledge in the present of the self or of the world which helps us to act intelligently.

However, the expression "I love Mary" can be more than an internal perception, for it can represent the outcome of a cognitive process. It can be a shorthand statement of "I know that I love Mary," with different consequences from a mere perceptual one. The discussion of this cognitive aspect will be postponed.

Let us now attempt to understand how self, perception, and object work together in life. But first I shall describe a laboratory experiment of Duncker's[1] that leads to the core of my views on perception. A subject stands in the middle of a striped rotating cylinder. Two different perceptions, either inward or outward bound, occur depending on the directive to the subject. If he is told to gaze at a spot on the striped, moving cylinder, he feels that he is moving and the cylinder is at rest. But if he is not given any directive, he perceives himself at rest and the cylinder as moving. In this experiment, perception gives knowledge either of self *or* of object (cylinder), not of both simultaneously.

It may be objected that the subject's perception of himself as rotating and the cylinder at rest is not a veridical perception. But a perception is a perception whether veridical or not. One might just as well label incorrect reasoning as not reasoning. Second, limiting the perceptual framework to either the subject or the cylinder and excluding the room where the experiment takes place, one can correctly state that either the subject is moving relative to the cylinder or the cylinder is moving relative to the subject. And, of course, the directive to gaze at a spot on the cylinder removes the room as a frame of reference for defining movement. The reference frame then becomes the cylinder or the body, and *either* the body *or* the cylinder is perceived as moving with reference to the other.

Let us turn now from the laboratory to an example from life: "I perceive Mary over there," and inquire whether here, too, only alternating knowledge of either self or object is achieved, as it is in the experiment.

The brief statement, "I perceive Mary," appears simple and unambiguous, but it isn't. It can have one of two meanings. In the one, "Mary" can be in the center of awareness in the sense that it is Mary I see and not Jane, Charlotte or a shadow or whatever. The "I see" is then on the periphery of awareness. The second meaning emphasizes *"I see"* with "I see" in the center of awareness and Mary in the periphery. This meaning could occur in the following way: "I see Mary, do you?" or in tests of visual acuity as "*I see* this line on the chart."

Turning now to internal perception, we ask whether "I love Mary" gives the same alternating knowledge of self and object as external perception does. Insofar as the statement conveys only a *feeling* of love, it is clear, without repeating the above discussion, that either the object "Mary" or the self "I love" is in the center of awareness while the other is in the periphery.

Our discussion of "I see Mary" and "I love Mary" diminishes the distinction usually made between external and internal perception. The difference is based on what is usual, not on any difference in principle between the two. In external perception the *object* is usually stressed; in internal perception, the *self* is usually stressed.

To summarize our discussion of perception: perception gives present knowledge of either the present self or the present object. It cannot give knowledge simultaneously of both self and object. It is also unable to acquaint us with the persisting identity in time and space of self and object. Such simultaneous knowledge of persisting identities of self and object is achieved only by the cognitive self, as will be discussed later on.

Corresponding to this alternating nature of perceptual knowledge of self and object are the syndromes of depersonialization and derealization. Similarly, this alternation of perceptual knowledge corresponds to the clinical fact that either one syndrome or the other appears, never both simultaneously (as far as I have observed). The source of these syndromes is to be found, I believe, in regression from the cognitive self to the perceptual self in an individual whose perceptual activity ordinarily occurs within a universe (a framework) established by the cognitive self. It may be imagined that perception pulses to and fro from self to object, attempting to achieve a synthesis of both. Its failure to achieve this synthesis results in the syndrome of unreality.

Now we have to look into the actual content of the assumed regression from the cognitive self to the perceptual self. We know what we mean by libidinal regression – a change in the aim of the drive with manifold alternations in the life of the individual. But what do we specifically mean by the abstract formula, regression from cognitive to perceptual self?

In order to uncover this specific meaning, we must finally turn to a discussion of the cognitive self. Let us turn back to the simple statement, "I love Mary." As already mentioned, it can be a statement of a *feeling* of love. As such, it is a mere perception. But it can also mean: "I finally am certain that I love Mary" or "I know that I love Mary." With this meaning, the statement becomes a cognitive one.

The consequences of each statement, perceptual or cognitive, are very different from each other, for feelings are transient and can come and go without necessarily altering life in a profound way. For example, the expression, "I feel hungry," is of immediate significance, but does not usually carry with it great potential for the future alteration of life. Of course, the statement of feeling love is more complex than that of feeling hunger, but still its implications (as only feeling) are of merely transient alterations of existence. Falling in and out of love in adolescence and at times in later life (i.e., in and out of feelings of love) is well known and only ripples the surface of existence.

But the consequences of the cognitive statement, "I love Mary," in the full sense (more than a mere perception of a feeling of love) are profound and enduring. An analysand at the beginning of his analysis was uncertain whether he loved his wife. When he finally came to the conclusion that he did, not only did his attitude toward her change, but also toward children and toward his career as well.

Let us look more thoroughly into this achievement of the patient and consider how (if not why) this patient improved in analysis, an area of psychoanalysis that continues to demand investigation.

For a long time the patient vacillated in his feelings toward his wife and given the framework within which he thought, he could come to no conclusion. At times he found her understanding, loving, delightful and at other times the opposite, and oscillated from one conclusion to the opposite one. Our goal is to ascertain how he achieved a definitive position.

Of course, we immediately think that his feelings became less ambivalent and more steadily positive. And this progress can be viewed as the consequence of an unknotting of libidinal fixations – fixations which had resulted from earlier unresolved unconscious conflicts.

But there is more than this to his achievement of a new position in life. The resolution of unconscious conflicts had only made it possible for him to achieve a new position. It did not lead him to it. Now we must attempt to follow those steps which led to it.

In his old position, his wife was an object of his drives. Insofar as she satisfied these drives, he had a positive position toward her, and insofar as she frustrated them, a negative one. During this period of his analysis, one aspect of his wife satisfied the classic definition of a drive; that which discharges it. With regard to his self, she was an object only insofar as his self was identified with a perceiving self, a self whose content was that of feelings released by perception of her. The object, his wife, had no existence beyond that of being a perceived object for the perceptual self.

In the course of analysis, the idea of the object became a constituent of his self. The thought of life without the object became intolerable because this loss was felt to be a contraction of self while life with her was felt to be an expansion of self. But, even with his new position, the patient still felt the same varying emotions toward his wife as part of his self. He was under no illusion that further analysis would produce a "blessed state" of unvarying feelings of love. His essential achievement consisted then in the simultaneous embracing of both the object and his perception of his varying feelings (his transient perceptual selves) by a higher one – the cognitive self. This was the basis of his achievement of a definitive position in life. This widening of the self seems to be one of the chief achievements of therapeutic analysis.

The difference between the mere perception of a feeling of love for Mary and the conclusive thought, "I finally know that I love Mary," lies in the unification achieved through cognition. The cognitive self embraces both the perception of the feeling of love (the perceptual self) and the object, Mary. The cognitive self owns both the object and the feeling of love and within that unity it still maintains the distinction of self (perceptual self) and object. To facilitate understanding, one can visualize a triangle: at the vertex lies the dominant, embracing conitive self; while the two angles at the base represent the object and the perceptual self.

This triangle constitutes a universe organized by the cognitive self, a universe in which the distinctions of perceptual self and object are marked off, and yet united. Imagine now the disappearance of the cognitive self from whatever cause. What is left is merely a perceptual system, with the perceptual self giving alternating knowledge of object and itself. This fluctuation of perception between the two is a condition, I believe, for the feeling of unreality in an individual in whom the more highly organized cognitive system had been dominant.

The return of the cognitive self and the consequent restablishment of a universe of object and perceptual self under its authority, puts an end to the feeling of unreality. Thus, Freud's feeling of unreality on the Acropolis[3] ended with the cognitive statement: "So all that really exists just as we learned it in school." This cognitive statement is characterized by a synthesis of present knowledge of the present ("So all that really exists") with present knowledge of the past ("as we learned it in school.").

With this cognitive act, the familiar stable world of things (e.g. the Acropolis, in this case) persisting in time reappeared. I believe that before this occurred, perception had freed itself from the embrace of cognition and had produced a world of merely momentary things and therefore an unreal world for Freud.

Not only had the stable world of things momentarily disappeared, but the persisting unity of the self in time had gone, too. "Just as we learned it in school" represents a binding of the self which in youth had first learned about the Acropolis with the self which now beheld it. This affirmation of the cognitive self shows that in a preceding moment, the unity of the self in time had vanished and been replaced by a purely present perceptual self. So we note that although Freud felt only the unreality of the object (the Acropolis), his self was nonetheless affected, too. And I believe that this is always so. Even though the feeling of unreality is attached either to the outside world or to the self, nonetheless a simultaneous destruction of the universe of existing object world and self previously established by the cognitive self always occurs in the syndrome of unreality.

The perceptual self alone cannot permeate its perceptions with a feeling of reality. To achieve this feeling of reality, the cognitive self embracing both object "out there" and immediate self is necessary. And a cognitive self reaching beyond the present into the past and yet retaining the present is also a necessity for the feeling of reality. The universe of identities – of persisting self and object – which is the guarantor of psychic reality is alone *created* by the cognitive self.

Freud's loss of a feeling of reality resulted from the momentary destruction of his universe by an unconscious conflict. Further on we will see that such a destruction can also come about from mechanical interferene with a sensory system. A destruction of this kind is usually transient except in the initial phase of schizophrenia. There the destruction of the world or of the self, alternately occupying the center of consciousness, lasts for some time. The return of a stable, persisting universe in schizophrenia is often achieved when the cognitive self accepts delusions about itself or the world.

The destruction of the universe of objects and the self (as persisting unities) in derealization and depersonalization demonstrates that these symptoms are very different from the usual neurotic one. They strike at the roots of existence, while the usual neurotic symptoms being circumscribed, leave most of the world and the self relatively untouched.

Why an unconscious conflict induces a profound regression from cognitive to perceptual self and gives rise to the syndrome of unreality in one case and in another does not induce such a regression, but gives rise only to the usual circumscribed neurotic symptom, cannot be ascertained with any degree of satisfaction. For example, it is not clear why Freud's unconscious conflict with his father gave rise to anxiety in his earlier years and later on to derealization. Numerous studies of the syndrome of unreality have demonstrated a number of factors, but none appears specific. The only suggestion I can offer (and it is far from satisfying) is that the very existence of the self and the world of objects may in some individuals be tied to a particularly vulnerable defense mechanism. In other cases, the cognitive self cannot maintain itself because the idea of the object must be extruded due to the quality of its cathexis. The self then tends to regress to a perceptual self, and existence becomes punctate. We have already alluded to this situation in the example with Tolstoy. He tried to meet the effects of this regression in an essentially child-like way. He hoped to feel good (internal perception) by doing good, and thus achieve a more continuous existence. His elaboration of this ethical philosophy need not concern us here.

In Freud's case, the reality of an inanimate "thing," the Acropolis, had been threatened by an internal conflict. Beside internal conflict, simple, external, mechanical interference with perception can threaten the reality of "things." Kohler's work with prism spectacles[7] demonstrates the similarity of mechanical interference and of mental conflict on the perception of the reality of the world of things.

The essence of Kohler's work (for us) is: the appearance of things is not merely altered by the use of prism spectacles, but the very existence of things is threatened, and the stability of the inanimate world, impaired. It is this aspect of his experimental work that makes it interesting for our discussion of self, perception, and object.

Before presenting a few of Kohler's findings, we must pause here and consider some of the attributes of a "thing" (in addition to its not being alive) that make it a "thing." For a "thing" to be a "thing," it must exist independently of me, and this independence is above all a spatial independence. For example, a thing must not ordinarily move when I move my head. If it does, I may polish my glasses to remove a speck of dust or dismiss the perception as an illusion caused by a floater in my eye. Second, a thing must usually have some consistency of shape; it cannot afford to be rubbery. This can be termed spatial identity. And finally it must possess an identity in time. How it appears today must be more or less its appearance tomorrow and the day after.

These attributes give us a world of stable, inanimate things in which we live with some confidence. But the wearing of prism spectacles destroys these attributes and, therefore, the world of inanimate things and our confidence in it.

The prism spectacles, it must be emphasized, do not merely alter the appearance of things; they destroy the spatial meaning of the usual world of things. But, better than this abstract discussion is a firsthand account of the effect of prism spectacles, and now I quote from Kohler:

"Writing about these first impressions in retrospect does not do them justice. The experience (i.e., of prism spectacles) is most uncanny. You are walking along, not worrying about a thing, since you can clearly see which way the street ahead of you goes. Then, all of a sudden, you know something is wrong. You could swear some mysterious force is trying to play a mean trick on you by always changing everything around at the last moment. . . . You get to the point where you cannot take anything for granted any more. [My underlining: note loss of confidence in things.] It is not your vision you blame, though; far from it; your confidence in your vision has not been shaken a bit by all this. No, it is the world you blame, the world whirling at your feet, which is trying to make a fool out of you. As for the apparent movements (this is a reference to movement of things when the subject moves his head), why should I think that they originate 'inside of me' rather than 'outside'? After all, don't they make the world look as if it were being shaken up by one earthquake after another? This is what makes those first impressions so unique.

"Shapes, too, change according to whether they are seen from above or below. A wall to my right arches over toward me; a wall to my left recedes from me. . . . "

In the course of wearing prism glasses, a further astonishing change occurs. Acute and obtuse angles again become verticals and horizontals; things lose their rubberiness and they no longer move when the subject moves his head. Despite continuing to wear the same prisms, the world of things finally becomes normal and stable, and the subject again regains confidence in it. A still further astonishing event occurs when the subject removes his prism spectacles and views the world once more with his normal glasses. Again, the stable world is lost for awhile, and all that disturbed him when he first wore the prism glasses now reappears when he is using his own. In time, this disturbance, too, disappears and the stable world redevelops.

These remarkable findings can be summarized as the result of a tendency toward stability. But such a tendency should not be considered as a finalistic, inexplicable principle; it is merely a capsular description.

What has actually happened toward the end of these remarkable experiments is that the cognitive self has finally achieved a new spatial system in which perception of the subject's body (perceptual self) and perception of the world of inanimate things (the objects) have been *achieved simultaneously*. This new spatial system replaces the one destroyed by either wearing or removing the spectacles.

Without in any way diminishing the beauty and importance of Kohler's work, contemplation of it removes our astonishment and tells us that that is the way the experiments should have turned out. We know that we see things right side up despite the inverted retinal image, and that Australians do not suffer from dizziness because "their heads are down," as we first thought when we learned about the other side of the globe. The world of objects that we see exists, of course, independently of us. But the way we see "things" (right-side-up, despite an inverted retinal image) results from the unitary spatial system of body and thing established by the cognitive self.

Not only the way we see things, but the way our body itself is experienced depends too on a similar spatial system. Just as the stability of the world of things is achieved by the creation of a spatial system harmonizing things and body, so the stability of the body itself depends on the establishment of a cognitive spatial system harmonizing body and things. So in drug states, the exclusion of the external world results in swellings and distortions of the body. The body loses its identity as a shape because of the loss of a universe organized into self and object. And the enlargement of after-images with increasing distance from the perceiver and their movement when the head moves are manifestations of their being narcissistic phenomena excluding the object.[7]

Kohler's experiments demonstrate that loss of a cognitive spatial system results in a transient, unstable, evanescent world. Stability of the world of things returns with the establishment of a spatial system embracing the perception of one's own body (self) and the external object – an achievement of the cognitive self.

This ever-widening embrace of the cognitive self may perhaps be one of the critical achievements of therapetuic psychoanalysis. It is represented unhappily by the tautological phrase "emotional insight." At first, the patient may respond to an "idea" (i.e. an interpretation offered by the analyst) with "I can see that, but I don't feel it." Again, this is unhappily called "intellectual insight." It is really only an example of the patient's capacity to follow inferences, but does not constitute insight. It is only knowledge. Nonetheless, it is worthwhile insofar as it demonstrates the intellect's relative freedom from conflict.

The interpretation remains an idea "out there." It remains an object that does not belong to the patient; it is not his. In the course of analysis, the "idea" silently and mysteriously becomes his. The cognitive self becomes enlarged through possessing the additional content, the interpretation. Making the idea *his* idea appears to be an outcome of working through. Numerous encounters with the idea show that the idea is true *for him,* not merely for the analyst. This being true for him is the result of a process in time, a connecting of the idea to the cognitive self. Stretching over time, the process of working through produces the unity of self and idea.

But how do numerous encounters with the object, "the idea" (the interpretation) show him that the idea is true for him? Numerous encounters in themselves could simply repeat the original intellectual encounter and therefore not contribute to a feeling of conviction. To be even a bit true for the analysand means that a feeling arises which is perceived – the perceptual self perceives its own inner state. We are thus back to our familiar triangle. The dominant vertex of the triangle – the cognitive self embraces the two bases, the interpretation (the external object) and the momentary feeling (the perceptual self). Then the analysand can say, "Yes, that is true."

Ultimately, the interpretation loses its separate existence as object and sinks into the obscurity of the self. It influences the analysand as automatically as our automatically absorbed horizontals and verticals guide our movements. Therefore, the analysand can only recover vague memories of various phases of his analytic work.

If the above description is accused of not really explaining the sense of conviction finally attached to the interpretation and its ultimate absorption into the self, the criticism must be accepted. But, if the criticism also implies that this ultimate mystery of analysis (the conviction of the truth of interpretation and the consequent growth of the self) is unique to psychoanalysis, then this implication must be rejected. The acceptance and rejection of new truths in the physical and biological sciences are by no means dependent only on their validity, just as it isn't in psychoanalysis. It usually takes time for an idea to be incorporated into these sciences. The acceptance of "the idea" in any science depends on making the system coherent with the new idea. How the sense of conviction develops is as clear or as mysterious in the physicobiological sciences as it is in psychoanalysis.

In using "self" throughout this paper, I may be confronted with the question, why not "ego." I will say right off that faced by the clinical material that stimulated this paper, I have used "self" instinctively. Of course, it is necessary to justify this instinctive position.

First of all, self emphasizes the present living experience and this has been the focus of my paper. The word "self" refers to the "I" of daily life as it occurs in the sentence "I went to the post office to buy stamps." Obviously, ego cannot be substituted for this "I" (although in German *"Ich"* can be used for either self or ego, a fact which has complicated our understanding of Freud.) Second, the universe under discussion consists of selves and objects, not of ego and objects. As Hartmann has pointed out,[5] the correlative to object is not ego, but self.

Finally, the primary phenomena consist in the self's experiences. Certainly in therapeutic work, we are interested in experience as the first plane on which our attention fixes. The self's experience is *the* phenomenon and the ego is secondary to this phenomenon and exists only as a construction for understanding it. The relation of self to ego is complex and awaits much fuller discussion than can be achieved within the scaffolding of this paper.[6]

The analysis of Freud's visit to the Acropolis and of Kohler's experiments appears to show that identity of inanimate things and identity of self are necessarily bound to each other. Since the Acropolis in Freud's unconscious conflict appears to represent a projection of his father and perhaps of his mother,[4] we can assume that identity of animate objects and identity of self are also tied to each other.

Exclusion of persisting identities of self and object in order to achieve a vivid sense of present reality (whether through drugs or a life of disconnected "happenings" must founder. The sense of present living reality is achieved only through transcending the present by the cognitive self which embraces the present and past experience and the external object.

Perhaps those moments of seeming vision into the very nature of the universe (experienced in particular in adolescence) are effects of momentary abolition of the cognitive self. They are characterized by a paradoxical sense of timeless eternity and of the immediate present (as in *déjà-vu*), pointing to a loss of identity in time.

We can only experience a stable world of objects (one of persisting identities in time and space) by possessing a similar identity of self. Similarly, we can only experience a persisting identity of self by possessing a stable world of persisting objects. To possess an existence stretching out in time, an identity, we must *create* it through cognitive activity. And cognitive activity can be taken as that activity of the mind which embraces both the object "out there" and the transient, perceptual self, and while remaining in the present, also reaches into the past.

References

1. Duncker, K. 1929. Über induzierte Bewegung. Psychl. Forschung, XII.
2. Freud, S. 1915. Instincts and their Vicissitudes. Standard Edition **14**: 117–140. Hogarth Press. London. 1957.
3. Freud, S. 1936. A Disturbance of Memory on the Acropolis. Standard Edition **22**: 239–248. Hogarth Press. London. 1964.

4. HARRISON, I. B. 1966. A Reconsideration of Freud's "A Disturbance of Memory on the Acropolis" in Relation to Identity Disturbance. Journal of the American Psychoanalytic Association **14**: 518–527. International Universities Press. New York.
5. HARTMANN, H. 1950. Comments on the Psychoanalytic Theory of the Ego. The Psychoanalytic Study of the Child **5**: 74–96. International Universities Press. New York.
6. JACOBSON, E. 1964. The Self and the Object World. International Universities Press. New York.
7. KOHLER, I. 1951. The Formation and Transformation of the Perceptual World. Psychological Issues, **3**(No. 4): 90–91. International Universities Press. New York.
8. SPIEGEL, L. A. 1959. The Self, The Sense of Self, and Perception. Psychoanalytic Study of the Child, **14**: 81–109. International Universities Press. New York.

Discussion

DR. PRAHM: Before I ask my question of Dr. Spiegel, I should like to bring something to the attention of Dr. Henderson which I meant to say before. This is in line with the argument Dr. Harms raised. I would say, in trems of Helmholtz's work, partcularly on the color perception, and since this was done by someone who was quoted repeatedly by Dr. Henderson, that he might like to know that the experiential position against the physiological and deterministic position of Helmholtz was particularly defended by Gurger, who is not quoted as a scientist too often, but is actually one of the percursors of modern theory of perception.

Regarding Dr. Spiegel's paper, I wonder whether he might elaborate a little on the differentiation between depersonalization and derealization, as he sees it.

DR. SPIEGEL: The overall term to be used is unreality. This syndrome is then divided into either depersonalization or derealization. In the former, the individual feels himself to be unreal. In the latter, he feels the external world to be unreal.

CHARLES HARRIS (*Bell Telephone Laboratories*): I think Dr. Spiegel might be interested in some recent experimental work following up on Ivo Kohler's experiments that I think brings out the other side of the coin that he was referring to. Dr. Spiegel, you were stressing that experiences of stability of the world and stability of the self are closely related.

The examples that you gave from Kohler's report had to do primarily with stability of the world, but in these recent experiments there has been some striking examples of how the same kinds of visually distorting prism glasses can lead to some quite strange perceptions of the self, and parts of the self. As an example: You put on right angle prisms that reverse the visual field into it's mirror image, as Kohler did, and then instead of simply going out into the world as he did and trying to adjust to this strange environment, you restrict yourself to a laboratory situation, where all that you see through the glasses is your own hand, and you try to write with that hand. Not only does one initially have difficulties doing this, as you'd expect, but most people would say that the hand that they're seeing is not a real hand; it's not moving the way they want it to.

Within a period of about 15 minutes many people would say that they see the hand, see it doing exactly what they feel it doing, that it's now fairly easy to write and work with this hand. However, what's intriguing about this is that again, contrary to the case that you referred to, you can demonstrate that what has happened here is not that the visual world has been turned around to agree with the feelings of the self, but rather that the kinesthetic feeling of the hand has been turned around to agree with the world.

With a revised visual world, and this you demonstrate by simply blindfolding the person and telling him, for example, to print some letters as you call them out. Very often, in fact something like a third of the time, he will either write the letter backwards and say that he feels he is writing a perfectly normal letter the way he's always written them. Or equally often he will write the letter correctly and he will say, that he felt I wrote it backwards. And carrying this further without going into the details, it seems as if in many of these experiments of Kohler's and other people, what happens and what underlies the apparently visual changes that you were referring to are actually what you might call kinesthetic, or proprioceptive changes in how the person experiences the parts of his body moving and where they are located in relation to other parts.

DR. SPIEGEL: Thank you very much for bringing this new data to my attention. It seems to me that these remarkable findings might be understood by applying the concept of postural schema. Furthermore, the alternating nature of perception, as suggested in this paper, might also be applicable to these data. Then either the rest of the body or the hand would function as a zero point.[8] (adaptation level of Helson)

PERCEPTION—YESTERDAY, TODAY, AND TOMORROW

Ernest Harms, Ph.D.

In my introductory remarks I mention Herman von Helmholtz as the greatest name in all perception studies. Helmholtz's greatness lay not only in the volume and depth of his work, but also in the breadth of his aspects and the objectivity he applied to the matters with which he had to deal. He attempted to cover the entire field, and in so trying, could not have failed to come across one of the most voluminous works on the theory of vision, J. W. v. Goethe's *Farbenlehre* (The Perception of Color). Goethe's work was never taken seriously, from a scientific point of view, in his own time and even less so afterwards. Helmholtz, however, did take it seriously. At the start of his career in 1853, he published a 30-page study on "Goethe's natural scientific works." Helmholtz rejected Goethe's basic theory but nevertheless he presented it with remarkable objectivity and compared it with his own point of view. Accordingly, Goethe, the genius with a poetical conception, was, in our language, a phenomenologist and existentialist who rejected speculative explanations and theories which reach beyond actual perception or the theory of sense perception. He demanded that our theories be found by the perceptive process. Goethe once wrote that "nature reveals all its secrets if we make the right effort to find them." Helmholtz agreed that Goethe was right insofar as his concepts can be applied. However, he placed these concepts against the inductive method which sees in the sense perceptions only signs for what lay behind them. They are symbols, like the written or spoken word, with which we identify reality. This, as we know, is the approach of all science, particularly natural science. Helmholtz admirably presented the two points of view or approaches which stand side by side but are opposed to one another. This was how Helmholtz saw himself at the start of his scientific career.

Throughout his career, Helmholtz struggled with Goethe's approach, and he mentioned him frequently. This fact comes clearly to the fore in his "Handbook of Physiological Optics" of 1867 which, without any doubt, is his most outstanding and most mature work. He discusses Goethe's approach repeatedly. In the chapter in which he sums up the history of optics, he says, about Goethe's *Farbenlehre,* that "the facts described are exactly observed, vividly described, and there cannot be any doubt about their correctness."

The most impressive aspect of this never-acknowledged relationship between Goethe's works and Helmholtz is that two years before his death in 1892, Helmholtz presented another paper about Goethe which he entitled "Goethe's Anticipation of Future Natural Science Ideas." He went into great detail regarding Goethe's phenomenological poetic creative process and how he applied it in his scientific studies of nature, which Helmholtz considered completely consequent. However, he still claimed that for a proper insight into the forces which motivate nature, one must apply the symbolic method of inductionalism. He closed with a reference to "Faust," in which Goethe deals with the theistic metaphysical experiences and speaks of the *Geheimnis,* (The Secret) which only the symbol can reveal. In this way, Helmholtz tried to justify his own magnificent work about the wider range of perceptual experience.

During his unique presentation of the physiology of human vision in his "Handbook of Optiks," Helmholtz suddenly comes forward with the amazing confession that in the final analysis physiology does not give us the final insight into human vision which he considered basically a *psychological* matter. In the middle of his 800-page volume, we find a chapter attempting an approach to the psychological problems of vision.

At first, however, Helmholtz claimed that no one in his time knew anything about the psychological process as applied to vision, that we therefore could actually know nothing about our sense perception; and he then referred to the future. However, leaving his actual inductive method behind, he attempted, so to speak, in a phenomenological, quite unmethodological, description of what he thought occurred concretely in any process of seeing. There are three "moments," he claims, in the psychological processes involved. First, the *Sinnes Empfindung,* in present terminology, "the Sensation," the impression made from outside upon our senses; second, the *Beobachtung* or the observation of the impression; and third, the *Deutung* or *Auslegung* or the interpretation which finally makes a perception complete. This important presentation by Helmholtz has not, up to now, been utilized by anyone.

When I was a student, the struggle in Helmholtz's mind occupied me considerably, but it has not been until recently that I have found the time to go back and research the matter.

Let me exemplify the Helmholtz insight in our language: First, I stand by my window looking down on the street. Suddenly, an unusual sensation touches my eye. I become alert. What is it? My observation as a second action gets under way: "That is a strong red color." And then a third conceptional action will be added: "Oh, that is a red dress on a woman." The perception is completed. Or another: A sensation of a sound touches my ear; next, observation sets in. "It is not the cry of a baby or an auto horn. I hear la, la, la, laaaa." "That is music, a bar of music." Then comes the third step, the memory-conception function. "That is the first bar of a Beethoven symphony." Not until now is the perception completed. It is one of our hopes here to bring forth the thesis that we must get away from the unreal sense-perceptional concept for explaining all perceptions. We must arrive at a differential and multiple concept. This concept must be basic for every kind of perception able to be applied to all in whatever field they appear. However, there is another aspect which I have taken the liberty of presenting in this paper. Namely, in Helmholtz's view there is one basic psychological concept that is actually valid for all perceptions. It claims that each perception is not a single unified psychological act, but a process composed of three psychological functions for which I have formulated these terms: *awareness, assertion,* and *perceptional conception**. A great deal of experimental and speculative work needs to be done in order to bring these facts up to the niveau of our present scientific demands. I hope that this presentation will initiate a new and fruitful development of our understanding and our knowledge of the most basic, most important, and most complicated of our psychological functions.

* Dr. Harry Helson, in the chapter on perception in his book Theoretical Foundations of Psychology (New York, 1951) points out that perception is not a simple factor, but is first completed when its adaptation level is reached. This concept goes clearly in the direction of the three functions in the perception process outlined here.

Part III. Perception in Abnormal Psychological Experience

ROLE OF PERCEPTION IN IDENTIFYING PSYCHOPATHOLOGY

Maurice Lorr, Ph.D.
Catholic University, Washington, D. C.

The process involved in the perception of psychopathology is relatively complex. On the one hand, the stimulus object or individual patient emits certain behaviors. Upon inquiry, or voluntarily, he also reports on inner states, attitudes, experiences, and discomforts labeled complaints. On the other hand the perceiver not only has his own frailties to deal with but also must interact with a moving, changing object. Kreitman[6] and Beck,[1] in their studies of rater errors, find omissions or failures to observe a comparatively important variable. Other errors are misperceptions of behaviors and distortions in the direction of the general impression evoked by the patient. Inference also plays an important role in distorting what is perceived and reported. Careful studies have shown that the rater who uses manifest phenotypic behavior as the primary basis for judgment is far less likely to make errors than one who employs inference primarily.

This leads one naturally to consider the role of training, experience, and implicit personality theory on perception and judgment. Can we properly infer that a syndrome obtained from an analysis of surface relations among attributes will necessarily yield a source of influence? Or do syndromes correspond to conventional concepts implied by the words the rater uses in making ratings?[16] For some obvious symptoms such as tics, bizarre postures, or hallucinations, there is little doubt. These behaviors are sufficiently discontinuous and deviant from normal behavior that it is unlikely that the rater could be misled by the language he used. However, in judging the presence of attributes relating to, say, hostility, anxiety, or dependency, the possibility of finding mere semantic factors or syndromes is very real indeed. An implicit conceptual framework or personality theory can impose itself on perception and judgment. Thus safeguards are needed to be sure that distinct concepts or constructs refer to internal structural characteristics of persons and not to semantic clusters.

Syndrome Identification

The question now is what psychotic and neurotic syndromes have been identified in current behavior by the method of factor analysis? Secondly, how closely do these statistically derived syndromes agree with those identified by clinicians. It should be noted immediately that the psychiatric diagnoses listed in the Manual[3] are in part based on current symptomotology and in part on life history variables. Important criteria are age, type of onset, precipitating events, course of illness, and recurrency. Thus a close correspondence between the two approaches should not be expected.

A syndrome is basically a statistical concept. It represents a highly correlated set of symptoms, behaviors, or complaints that is independent of other observable symptom complexes. When a clinician identifies a syndrome on the basis of his observations of a sample of patients, he is engaging in an arm-chair form of factor analysis. He detects a functional unity and gives it a name. The statistical procedure of factor analysis is simply a more rigorous way of examining the similarities within a large set of symptoms. The computer first estimates the degree of similarity between each and every symptom noted. Then it isolates each relatively unique and independent grouping within the correlations between the symptoms.

Attention will now be turned to a description and summary of the syndromes thus far isolated from behavioral observations. They represent, of course, the perceptual unities of the observer which, hopefully, correspond to existing behavioral unities in patients.

The Minor Psychotic Syndromes

The groupings perceived by clinicians will be referred to as syndromes since they conform to the common meaning of the term (see TABLE 1). Each represents a cluster of symptoms, behaviors, and complaints that tend to occur together with high frequency. They will be referred to as "minor" syndromes to distinguish them from the major disorders.

The studies to be reported all utilized the Inpatient Multidimensional Psychiatric Scale (IMPS). This rating schedule is designed to measure 12 psychotic syndromes confirmed in repeated factor analyses.[13] IMPS consists of 89 brief rating scales and dichotomous items. Ratings are made following interviews of 30 to 45 minutes in length.

Each syndrome is defined by a set of scales, from 5 to 11 in number, that measure a unitary pattern of behavior. The labels given the syndromes are intended to describe the underlying response tendency. For convenience in referral each syndrome is also identified by three letters. The 12 syndromes are briefly characterized as follows:

Excitement (EXC): The patient's speech is hurried, loud, and difficult to stop. His mood level and self-esteem are elevated and his emotional expression tends to be unrestrained or histrionic. He is also likely to exhibit controlling or dominant behavior.

Hostile Belligerence (HOS): The patient's attitude toward others is one of disdain and moroseness. He is likely to manifest much hostility, resentment, and a complaining bitterness. His difficulties and failures tend to be blamed on others.

Paranoid Projection (PAR): The patient gives evidence of fixed beliefs that attribute a hostile, persecuting, and controlling intent to others around him.

Grandiose Expansiveness (GRN): The patient's attitude toward others is one of superiority. He exhibits fixed beliefs that he possesses unusual powers. He reports divine missions and may identify himself with well-known or historical personalities.

Perceptual Distortions (PCP): The patient reports hallucinations (voices and visions) that threaten, accuse, or demand.

Obsessional-Phobic (OBS): The patient reports compulsive acts and rituals, recurrent obsessive thoughts, specific phobias, and ideas of depersonalization and change.

Impaired Functioning (IMP): Patients complain of inability to make decisions, to concentrate, and to work. They also report a loss of interest in people, sex, and social activity.

Anxious Depression (ANX): The patient reports vague apprehension as well as specific anxieties. His attitudes toward himself are disparaging. He is also prone to report feelings of guilt and remorse for real and imagined faults. The underlying mood is typically dysphoric.

Retardation and Apathy (RTD): The patient's speech, ideation, and motor

TABLE 1

THE MINOR PSYCHOTIC SYNDROMES
BRIEF DESCRIPTIONS OF BEHAVIORS PRESENT

Excitement (EXC)

7. Unrestrained emotionality
9. Hurried speech
12. Elevated mood
17. Dramatization
20. Loud speech
26. Overactivity
37. Excess speech
40. Dominating

Hostile Belligerence (HOS)

5. Verbally hostile
11. Contemptuous
18. Attitude hostile
25. Irritable
28. Blaming others
32. Bitter
36. Complaining
38. Suspicious

Paranoid Projection (PAR)

50. Delusional
73. Ideas of reference
74. Ideas of persecution
75. Delusions of conspiracy
76. People controlling
77. External controlling
82. Somatic delusions

Grandiosity (GRN)

15. Attitude of superiority
67. Voices extoll
78. Unusual powers
79. Great personality
83. Divine mission

Perceptual Distortion (PCP)

51. Hears voices
66. Voices accuse
68. Voices threaten
69. Voices order
70. Visions
71. Other hallucinations
81. Ideas of change

Obsessional-Phobic (OBS)

47. Obsessive thoughts
48. Phobias
49. Compulsions
72. Self-change
81. Environmental change

Anxious Depression (ANX)

14. Blaming self
21. Specific anxiety
24. Apprehension
27. Self-depreciating
29. Depressed
31. Guilt feeling
43. Shows insight
46. Suicidal
80. Sinful

Impaired Functioning (IMP)

59. Indecisive
60. Unable to concentrate
61. Fatigued
62. Lacking interest
63. Can't get started
64. Lacking sex interest

Retardation (RTD)

1. Slowed speech
8. Lacking goals
13. Fixed facies
16. Slowed movements
19. Memory deficit
22. Speech blocking
23. Apathy
30. Slovenly
33. Whispered speech
41. Failure to answer

Disorientation (DIS)

84. Re hospital
85. Re state
86. Knows no one
87. Re season
88. Re year
89. Re age

Motor Disturbances (MTR)

6. Bizarre posture
10. Motor tension
52. Giggling
53. Grimacing
54. Repetitive movements
57. Talks to self
58. Startled glances

Conceptual Disorganization (CNP)

2. Irrelevant speech
3. Incoherent speech
4. Rambling speech
55. Neologisms
56. Stereotyped phrases

activity are delayed, slowed, or blocked. In addition, he is likely to manifest apathy and disinterest in the future.

Disorientation (DIS): The patient's orientation with respect to time, place, and season is defective. He may show failure to recognize others around him.

Motor Disturbances (MTR): The patient assumes and maintains bizarre postures, and he makes repetitive facial and body movements.

Conceptual Disorganization (CNP): Disturbances in the patient's stream of thought are manifested in irrelevant, incoherent, and rambling speech. Repetition of stereotypes phrases and coining of new words are also common.

The syndromes have been shown to be sufficiently reliable in a variety of settings.[12] Some of the evidence for the validity of the syndromes has been reported.[10] In brief, it has been shown that the syndrome scores are related to ward assignment, to prominent features of psychopathology, and to conventional diagnostic class membership. The syndromes have also been found to be sensitive to change with tranquilizer treatment and to psychopathology as determined by various measuring devices.

The Major Psychotic Disorders

The most recent edition of *Mental Disorders*[3] distinguishes three classes of functional disorders. The schizophrenics are identified principally by their thought disorders. The affective psychoses are characterized by disorders of mood that represent either extreme depression or elation. The paranoid states are distinguished from schizophrenia by narrow delusions and the absence of other symptoms. Each of the major disorders are defined both by life history data and by disturbances in current behavior, thinking, and mood.

Recent studies concerned with definition of the major psychotic disorders have been based on *currently* observable disturbances in thinking, mood, and behavior entirely. The minor syndromes, just described, tend to be correlated. When the correlations among the minor syndromes are analyzed by factor analysis, five more inclusive major syndromes or disorders can be demonstrated. There have been reports on the major disorders, using factor analysis, by Degan,[4] Lorr and colleagues,[13] Overall and colleagues,[18] Cohen and coworkers,[2] Lorr and coworkers,[11] and most recently by Lorr and Klett.[9] The five disorders identified are described in terms of the more elementary syndromes in the columns of TABLE 2. An asterisk implies that the minor syndromes are substantially correlated with the disorder listed at the top of the column. These disorders will now be described.

Disorganized Hyperactivity is defined by general excitement, conceptual disorganization, and to a lesser extent, by grandiosity and motor disturbances. Manic-depressive psychosis-manic type is clearly a close equivalent in terms of its behavioral characteristics.

Hostile Paranoia is characterized by paranoid delusions, hostile belligerence, and resistiveness. It is narrower than the other four major disorders, but it has appeared repeatedly in widely different data. There does not appear to be any equivalent disorder recognized by the APA diagnostic manual.

Psychotic Depression is defined primarily by anxious depression, functional impairment, and the obsessional-phobic syndrome. Evidently then, the affective disorders are represented by both *Disorganized Hyperactivity* and *Psychotic Depression.* It should be observed that the affective disorders depressive in character that are recognized in Mental Disorders differ primarily in social history. Involutional melancholia is associated with the involutional period. The

TABLE 2

THE MAJOR PSYCHOTIC DISORDERS AS DEFINED BY THE MINOR SYNDROMES

Minor Syndromes	Disorganized Hyper-activity	Hostile Paranoia	Psychotic Depression	Paranoid Process	Schizophrenic Disorganiza-tion
Excitement	+				
Hostile Belligerence		+			
Paranoid Projection		+		+	
Grandiosity	+			+	
Perceptual Distortion				+	
Obsessional-Phobic			+	+	
Anxious Depression			+		
Functional Impairment			+		
Retardation					+
Disorientation					+
Motor Disturbances	+				+
Conceptual Disorganization	+				+

manic-depressive variety is characterized by remission and recurrency. It is quite possible that the behavioral pattern is the same in various diagnostic classes.

The fourth disorder, *Paranoid Process,* is defined by paranoid delusions, grandiosity, hallucinations, and to a lesser degree, by obsessional thinking. The paranoid states do not appear to correspond to this disorder. The appearance of this broad dimension in a very wide range of studies indicates that the evidence is strong. The closest equivalent may be found in an increasingly popular subdivision of schizophrenia into the paranoid and nonparanoid.[5,21] The *Paranoid Process* may represent the dimension corresponding to paranoid schizophrenia.

The fifth disorder has been labeled *Schizophrenic Disorganization* because it corresponds so closely to the symptom pattern ordinarily characterized in nonparanoid schizophrenia. It is defined by retardation, disorientation, motor disturbances, and to a lesser extent, by conceptual disorganization. Patients scoring high on this dimension tend to be hospitalized longer and to have a longer history of a psychotic breakdown. It may be conjectured that the "process schizophrenic" is very likely to have his highest scores on this measure.

THE NEUROTIC SYNDROMES

The Manual of Mental Disorders[3] lists nine neurotic syndromes. These traditional diagnostic classes include anxiety, phobias, obsessive compulsions, depressions, hysteric conversion and disassociation, neurasthenia, hypochondriasis, and depersonalization. These symptom groupings originate in the clinic from observations of the clinician who notes the joint presence of certain complaints and behaviors. It is of some interest to contrast these with those derived by statistical means. As was noted earlier, arm-chair factor analysis is essentially the same as statistical factor analysis.

Numerous reports have long been available on self-report data stemming from analyses of the MMPI.[8,22,23] More recently the need for evaluating drug effectiveness has stimulated the development of various devices that utilize both psychiatric and patient reports. In addition to several[14] earlier studies by O'Connor,[17] there are reports by Raskin and his colleagues,[19,20] by Lipman and colleagues,[7] and by Mattsson and colleagues.[15] Fortunately there is good agreement between self-reported and observer-reported symptom groupings. The results have been organized and presented in TABLE 3.

Many of the traditional neurotic syndromes are found listed under the label of minor syndromes. Anxiety-Tension, Depression, Obsessive-Compulsive, and Somatic Complaints correspond closely to those classes long recognized. However, syndromes or factors such as Shyness, Hostile Feeling, Suspicion, and Autism (peculiar and unusual ideation) are not recognized as such. Perhaps this is because these disturbances are regarded as secondary phenomena to the more severe symptoms. Phobias usually are absorbed under Anxiety-Tension. Hysteric Conversion and Disassociation fail to appear simply because the study samples have not included appropriate cases. There is little doubt that these groups would emerge if broader samples were examined.

Clinicians and researchers have long recognized that the neurotic syndromes have much in common. This general tendency is represented in the hierarchical arrangement shown in TABLE 3. Factor analyses by Wiggins[23] and by Lorr[8] and Lorr and Rubenstein[15] have indicated both in observer and questionnaire data three "group" syndromes. These have been tentatively labeled Anxiety Proneness, Externalization and Impulsivity, and Somatic Concern.

Those who develop anxiety or depression and those who complain of social fear are most likely to be treated by psychotherapy in our clinics. On the other hand, persons reporting hostile feeling, suspicion, peculiar dreams and thoughts, and recurrent ideas are typically judged to be unsuited for psychotherapy. Indeed some may be regarded as having character disorders. By and large these tendencies imply externalization of blame and problems of impulse control. Somatic concern represents that large segment of neurotics with vague transient somatic complaints.

All of these symptom and complaint groupings have in common what may be called Neuroticism. This dimension represents a readiness to be disturbed, annoyed, or thrown off balance by stress and by threat, by both interpersonal and environmental sources. Further, the stronger the neurotic component, the longer the reaction is likely to persist.

TABLE 3

THE CONFIRMED MINOR SYNDROMES AND THEIR RELATION TO NEUROTICISM

Minor Syndromes	Group Syndromes	General Disorder
Anxiety-Tension	Anxiety	
Depression	Proneness	
Shyness		
Hostile Feeling		
Suspicion	Externalization	Neuroticism
Autism	& Impulsivity	
Obsessive-Compulsive		
Somatic Complaints	Somatic	
GI Complaints	Concern	

Another characteristic of some importance distinguishes the anxiety-prone from the externalizers and the somatic complainers. Those in the first group have insight into their conditions but are prone to ascribe a wide range of socially undesirable attributes to themselves. Those manifesting other syndromes tend to deny common frailties or any personal role in the problems they report.

Finally it is worth noting that the observer plays less a role as we move from the psychoses to the neuroses. The major source of evidence comes from manifest behavior in the psychotic disorders. Information on the neurotic conditions is gained primarily from patient self-reports supplemented by inferences from what the patient says about his views and attitudes towards others.

Discussion

The studies summarized show increasing convergence onto a limited set of descriptive categories of psychopathology. Observers of psychotic behavior identify 12 or so minor syndromes and five more inclusive patterns or disorders. Since there has been less research on the neurotic syndromes, agreement among researchers is not as great. The available evidence indicates that the more elementary syndromes combine into three more general patterns. Underlying all of these may be found a tendency towards neuroticism, on which everyone may be ranked as to degree.

Thus far the personality disorders have not been mentioned. In contrast with the psychotic and neurotic disorders, classification of the personality disturbances rests far more on social history, long-term observation and patient self-reports. In fact the role of self-report becomes increasingly important in appraisal, at least if the patient is to be evaluated within a few hours. This is the same as saying that the observer becomes less and less important as we move from the more severely to the less severely disturbed and disorganized. The interviewer simply repeats what the patient has told him. Or, he makes inferences regarding the individual's ego maturity, attitudes toward authority, self-concept, or other comparable matters.

Mention may also be made, for the sake of completeness, of other problems relating to the observation of psychopathology. First, how are impressions of a patient formed? Are attributes put together by some summation process involving the simple addition of items varying in magnitude? Or, as some contend, are attributes combined by averaging? The problem is obviously quite general and applies to all impression formation.

Another problem that has been investigated recently concerns judges' perception. Do judges or observers differ in cognitive complexity? The structure imposed by some observers may be much more complex than that evident in others. There is also the notion that everyone carries an implicit personality theory around with him. There may be subvarieties of implicit personality theories. Support for this contention may be found in the analysis of the concept of social desirability. Edwards has shown that people generally tend to report what is socially desirable about themselves. However, neurotics tend to report socially undesirable things about themselves. In fact Messick demonstrated that there may be as many as ten distinctive viewpoints of social desirability.

Classification on the basis of symptoms and behavior makes no explicit assumptions regarding etiological factors. However, it seems clear that the various syndromes are at least influenced by people and circumstances. Others might argue that they are in fact maintained or reinforced by these conditions. Assessment of a patient's behavior should, therefore, include an examination and evaluation of the significant other people and the environmental conditions in his life that appear to elicit various behaviors. In this manner environmental analysis might well yield a useful conceptual system of stimulus or situational dimensions that evoke deviant behavior.

References

1. Beck, A. T., *et al.* 1962. The reliability of psychiatric diagnoses: II. a study of consistency of clinical judgments and ratings. Amer. J. Psychiat. **119:** 351–357.
2. Cohen, J., *et al.* 1966 (Jan.) Dimensions of psychiatric symptom ratings determined at thirteen time points from hospital admission. J. Consult. Psychol. **30:** 39–44.
3. Committee on Nomenclature. 1968. Diagnostic and Statistical Manual of Mental Disorders. American Psychiatric Assoc. Washington, D. C.
4. Degan, J. W. 1952. Dimensions of functional psychosis. Psychometric Monographs, No. 6.
5. Johannsen, W. J., S. H. Friedman, T. H. Leitschuh & H. Ammons. 1963. A study of certain schizophrenic dimensions and their relationship to double alteration learning. J. Consult. Psychol. **27:** 375–382.
6. Kreitman, N., P. Sainsbury, J. Morrissey, J. Towers & J. Scrivner. 1961. The reliability of psychiatric assessment: an analysis. J. Ment. Sci. **107:** 887–908.
7. Lipman, R. S., K. Rickles, L. Covi, L. R. Derogates & E. H. Uhlenhuth. 1969. Factors of symptom distress. Arch. Gen. Psychiat. **21:** 328–338.
8. Lorr, M. 1968. A test of seven MMPI factors. Mult. Behav. Res. Special Issue : 151–156.
9. Lorr, M. & C. J. Klett. 1969. Major psychotic disorders: a cross-cultural study. Arch. Gen. Psychiat. **19:** 652–658.
10. Lorr, M. & C. J. Klett. 1966. Inpatient Multidimensional Psychiatric Scale Manual. Consulting Psychologist Press. Palo Alto, Calif.
11. Lorr, M., C. J. Klett & R. Cave. 1967 (Jan.) Higher-level psychotic syndromes. J. Abnorm. Psychol. **72:** 74–77.
12. Lorr, M., C. J. Klett, D. M. McNair & J. J. Lasky. 1962. Manual: Inpatient Multidimensional Psychiatric Scale. Consulting Psychologist Press. Palo Alto, Calif.
13. Lorr, M., C. J. Klett & D. M. McNair. 1963. Syndromes of Psychosis. Pergamon Press.
14. Lorr, M. & E. A. Rubinstein. 1956. Personality patterns of neurotic adults in psychotherapy. J. Consult. Psychol. **20:** 257–263.
15. Mattsson, N. B., *et al.* 1969. Dimensions of symptom distress in anxious neurotic outpatients. Psychopharmacology Bull. **5:** 19–32.
16. Mulaik, S. A. 1964. Are personality factors raters' conceptual factors? J. Consult. Psychol. **28:** 506–511.
17. O'Connor, J. P. 1953. A statistical test of psychoneurotic syndromes. J. Abn. Soc. Psychol. **48:** 581–584.
18. Overall, J. E., L. E. Hollister & P. Pichot. 1967 (Feb.) Major psychiatric disorders. Arch. Gen. Psychiat. **16:** 146–151.
19. Raskin, A., J. Schulterbrandt, N. Reatig & C. E. Rice. 1967. Factors of psychopathology in interview, ward behavior and self-report ratings of hospitalized depressives. J. Consult. Psychol. **31:** 270–278.
20. Raskin, A., M. S. Schulterbrandt, N. Reatig & J. J. McKeon. 1969. Replication of factors of psychopathology in interview, ward behavior and self-report ratings of hospitalized depressives. J. Nerv. Men. Dis. **148:** 87–98.
21. Shakow, D. & P. E. Huston. 1936. Studies of motor functions in schizophrenia: I Speed of Tapping. J. Gen. Psychol. **15:** 63–106.
22. Tryon, R. 1966. Unrestricted cluster and factor analysis with applications to the MMPI and Holzinger-Harmon problems. Mult. Behav. Res. **1:** 229–244.
23. Wiggins, J. S. 1966. Substantive dimensions of self-report in the MMPI item pool. Psychological Monographs, No. 630.

Discussion of the Paper

William McGarvey (*College at Oswego, the State University of New York*): I'm concerned over your continued use of the term "introversion" as one of the qualities that defines the maladjusted. Is there such a thing as a healthy introvert is essentially the question I'm putting to you.

DR. LORR: A better word might be social fear or shyness. Yes, I would say that a person, in keeping with jungian theory, would be within a normal range. I'm really talking about the embarrassment, or anxiety that's pathological.

MARTIN LINDAUER (*State University of New York at Brockport*): Some of us who call ourselves perception psychologists are concerned with the definition of perception. And for the most part we spend our energy I think separating perception from sensation, or from cognition, let's say. As I gather from your presentation, and perhaps from others as well in the preceding day, perception is applied extremely broadly to include personality variables and other dynamic factors. And I just wonder whether you think that perception can justifiably be treated so broadly? Or whether you share our concern with the more, closer more careful definition of the term "perception."

DR. LORR: I would say I agree. I think that possibly Dr. Harms could better answer this question. I might say that direct observation of external behavior and phenomena certainly comes within the general definition of what is perceived, and what one might regard as self-report as a form of internal perception. But I certainly wouldn't argue with you on your more rigorous and limited concept of the particular construct of perception.

PROF. MARY BLADE (*Cooper Union*): I wonder if you'd continue your comments about environmental analysis? You just hinted at it at the end.

DR. LORR: As an illustration we recently completed a study concerned with interpersonal behavior, and it's quite obvious that interpersonal behavior doesn't occur in a vaccum. The way typical questionnaires are handled, the stimulus situation is simply neglected or ignored, and so, utilizing incomplete sentences, we first collected stimuli and then responses in large samples. We were able to break up the interpersonal area on the combination of a stimulus and response. Here is an illustration: When my friend tells me what to do, my response may be that I get mad and tell him off, or I ignore him, or I feel hurt and walk away, or I do what he says. And so what we did was to analyze interpersonal patterns, and we actually found something like six dimensions of interpersonal stimuli related to control, nurturance, dependency, exclusion and hostility. So it was along these avenues that we were considering our research.

ARTHUR WILLNER (*Hillside Hospital*): There's an impression given from the structures that you've indicated, that they include all the possible syndromes that you find clinically. It seems to me that this is not particularly helpful. We've been able to isolate a syndrome, specifically phobic anxious depersonalization, which has been particularly helpful in treatment, especially in very specific drug treatment. This would seem to cut across some of the categories that you've indicated. If the samples that you included were larger, it would seem to me that it might very well alter the particular structures that you have elicited.

DR. LORR: I'm inclined to agree with you. For example, careful studies of restricted depressive groups disclose a syndrome called depressive mood. If you now include a large sample of all types of psychotics within your analysis, this particular pattern vanishes. And so I'm convinced, like yourself, that supplementary studies are needed of specialized groups. The structures, the patterns within those particular groups, like depressions, might well be much more complex than they are within a larger group.

CHANGING RELATIONS OF SYMPTOM PERCEPTION TO PSYCHOANALYTIC THERAPY

Benjamin Wolstein, Ph.D.

W. A. White Institute of Psychiatry, Psychoanalysis and Psychology, New York and Adelphi University, Garden City, N. Y.

The perception of symptoms and inquiry into their origins and functions acquired an important place very early in the history of psychoanalysis, going as far back as Breuer and Freud's 1895 Studies on Hysteria. Only recently, however, has it been recognized that becoming free of symptoms is not the same as becoming different psychologically. Psychoanalytic patients appear far less inhibited, today, than either early freudian id patients about sexual instinct functions or later freudian ego-interpersonal patients about adaptive social functions. Psychoanalytic patients now appear to suffer far less from unsatisfied biological needs and failed social securities than from blocked strivings for psychic freedom and personal fulfillment. In this paper, I consider some reasons why these extensions and enlargements came about.

In the crucial 1915–1917 Introductory Lectures, Freud remarked that the psychoanalytic task is to remove symptoms because that is what the patient actually seeks in undertaking the therapeutic effort. We must take note how far from this the field has developed; not only does the psychoanalyst no longer focus on removing symptoms but also the patient no longer expects it; and neither coparticipant pursues it as the main goal of therapeutic inquiry. For whatever else it is, and it is many other things, perception of symptoms is a profoundly social and cultural phenomenon – a mode of communication, symbolization, legitimation. Because this is so, what can be perceived and conceived as symptom requires the cooperation of other factors that help to symbolize it as symptom in the common knowledge of conventional wisdom. In this sense, a symptom serves as identifying credential in sociological terms: just as graduation from a training institute serves as social credential for the psychoanalyst's practice of this therapy, so certain symptoms serve as social credentials for the patient's entry into this therapy. Symptom perception is, then, a justifying condition for psychoanalytic inquiry – an initial condition, so to speak, communicating the patient's purpose in being in therapy, legitimating his desire to undertake the effort, relating and symbolizing processes and patterns of his life experience. There is nothing particularly new and unconventional about this point of view; it is even very well advertised, now, by the literary experts in pop culture. Recall, for a moment, Portnoy's long and windy 274-page effort to establish the validity of his complaint as psychoanalyzable symptom, involving his parents, friends, colleagues, and mistresses, as well as his self-hating masturbatory complex. It is only after he repeats it and his story beyond the point of boredom, it should be noted, that Dr. Spielvogel finally says, "So . . . Now vee may perhaps to begin. Yes?"

It is not necessary to set the order of precedence in each case, for therapeutic purposes, between changing perceptions of symptoms and changing models of psychoanalytic therapy. Without getting into the old chicken-egg twister of which came first, it is possible to put the changes schematically. In the id impulse model, symptom perception is biological and instinctual; in the ego-interpersonal model, symptom perception is social and cultural; in the model of shared experience, symptom perception is personal and psychological. It is probably clear, even from so brief a schema of the three major psychoanalytic models, that certain perceived symptoms legitimate certain therapeutic models by a two-way process moving back and forth between them. Some psychoanalysts not exclusively committed to any single metapsychology already began to sense this in the early 1950's, I believe, when they spoke rather loosely of this patient needing a freudian therapist, that one an adlerian therapist, another a jungian therapist, and so on; or, this is a freudian patient, that an adlerian patient, another a jungian patient, and so on – indirectly asserting the intimate connection among symptom perception, model of therapy and perspective on metapsychology. With symptom perception so varied, models of therapy so changing, perspectives on metapsychology so open and pluralistic, the need for order and clarity gave rise to a new interest in basic features common to all therapy distinctly psychoanalytic. Although it is a topic for another paper, I allude to this new significance of psychoanalytic structure subsequently. But I am mainly concerned, here, with reviewing the history of these changing relations of symptom perception to psychoanalytic therapy, and sketching a structure of inquiry presently underlying the three major models – id impulse, ego-interpersonal relation, and shared experience.

Three Models of Therapy

Even a brief historical outline of psychoanalysis over the past 75 years would indicate that changes in symptom perception went through three major models of therapy. They are: id impulse, ego-interpersonal relation, and shared experience. I generally select these for special attention because, first, Freud's id model from which Adler, Jung, and Rank later developed theirs was dominant until the middle 1920's; second, the ego-interpersonal model to which Reich, A. Freud, Hartmann, and Sullivan, among others, contributed was dominant from the middle 1930's onward; and third, since the radical and extensive clinical studies of transference, resistance, anxiety and counteranxiety, counterresistance, countertransference from the early 1950's to the present, the new model of shared experience has been in the making. This selected listing does not mean that, during the last 75 years, no variants of these models were ever practiced; nor does placing these three in historical sequence mean that other earlier ones are no longer practiced after the emergence of later ones. There is no doubt that variations of these models of id impulse, ego-interpersonal relation and shared experience have always existed; that others have always been, and still are being, practiced; and that psychoanalysts today may still work with any of the various earlier models. But these facts are, clearly, no more than footnotes to a historical sketch of the major changes and the major reasons for them in intelligible perspective.

It is not necessary, for these purposes, to go into great detail about the origins of these three models or about the distinguishing features of each one. The interested reader may find this information elsewhere.[1] It is only necessary, here, to consider some salient factors guiding the changes. Along the way from Freud's 1915–1917 design for id therapy to Reich's late 1920's innovation of character analysis leading to ego-interpersonal therapy, for example, there was the crucial observation that careful genetic study of affective experience alone does not suffice to free the patient's psychological growth in difficult and troubled periods of his life. For if psychic trauma is not simply an affair of the id, and if cognitive activity is also always in some sense present through all his difficulties and troubles, the psychoanalyst must treat his patient, then, as experiencing in both the affective and the cognitive modes. Now this may seem like a very simple proposition whose truth is practically self-evident. But it proved to have revolutionary implications for the established model of id therapy, bringing about irreversible changes in procedures and perspectives. Putting this in the terms of classical psychoanalytic therapy: without the ego there can be no study of the id.

Once the patient's ego was admitted into the classical model, however, and he could think openly about his inner problems in the experiential field of therapy, it was but a short step for him to admit the things he thinks about in his social life as well. And so he brought in ego-interpersonal insecurities in addition to id impulse frustrations or, more generally, questions about social goals, ego values and interpersonal relations in addition to problems of organ function and sexual intimacy. This change from the id impulse to the ego-interpersonal model was consolidated in the 1930's. And it was systematically instated as the adaptive point of view, or as the adjustment of organism and environment, man and culture, interpersonal relation and social order. In one variation or another, all ego-interpersonal models share this postulate of adaptation or adjustment. But is this notion, in principle, a matter of postulation? Is it not, rather, a theme of meta-psychology originally deriving from biological Darwinism and later penetrating into all forms of social and ego-interpersonal Darwinism? From the standpoint of psychoanalytic structure, that is, it rightfully belongs at the order of metapsychology as a matter of overall philosophic perspective, and not at the order of postulates or points of view introduced for empirical and systematic psychoanalysis of experience.

The change from both the id impulse and the ego-interpersonal models to that of shared experience is, therefore, an even further development. While id therapy works inward, so to speak, from psychic manifestations down into sources of impulse, and while ego-interpersonal therapy works outward, so to speak, from psychic manifestations up into social and cultural objectives of adaptation, therapy of shared experience works with psychic manifestations where and when they are, how and what they can become, whether and why they should be—all these, it may be emphasized, in the therapeutic field in which they are observed and defined, transformed and explained, interpreted and philosophized. This model represents a fresh effort in the history of psychoanalysis to deal with therapeutic experience as made up of psychological processes and patterns occurring under psychological conditions and treatable in psychologial terms, yet leaving interpretation of their contents and values to the individual metapsychologies of the particular coparticipants. The point is, psychoanalyst and patient are no longer hooked into any single metapsychology – freudian, adlerian, jungian, rankian, and so on, even, to ego-interpersonal adaptation – simply by virtue of their shared inquiry into their shared experience. Nor do they, in fact, require any prior commitments to any single metapsychology or value system in order to secure involvement in serious psychoanalytic inquiry. Relatedness and communication suffice as the basis of a factual account of human possibilities for psychoanalytic experience. For the coparticipants inevitably relating and communicating have no choice but to experience each other and, in doing so, have no choice but to assimilate and analyze this experience in the only ways they finally can.

As background for this change, we must recall again the salient factors guiding it. Along the way from Reich's character analysis, A. Freud's and Hartmann's ego psychology and therapy, and Horney's and Sullivan's cultural and interpersonal therapy of the 1930's, there was the crucial observation that transference did not take place in a psychological vacuum, to be studied by a neutral mirror or professional expert as though he himself were not actively present in the very field of experience in which he is involved. It was observed, indeed, that the psychoanalyst was actively present and coparticipating in the experiential field of therapy far more than a neutral mirror which reflected back only what was said to it, far more than a detached expert from whose clear point of view observations were made, and far more than a purveyor of any olympian metapsychology, of course, or any single value system exclusively. Not only his learned psychoanalytic procedures, but, in addition, his self, his persona, his very psyche are actively present and coparticipating in varied therapeutic fields with wide varieties of patient seeking therapeutic experience. And when it was also observed, in the 1950's, that transference did not occur as discrete process or isolated pattern but, instead, in functional relation to both resistance and anxiety, it was quite an easy step to combine the two observations. Thus, if transference does not take place in a mirrored vacuum or in the presence of a detached professional expert, then neither does the cluster of transference, resistance, anxiety. From here it is, again, quite a direct step to the psychoanalytic study of shared experience. Since the cluster of transference, resistance, anxiety is to be studied from the standpoint of the other coparticipant as well, then it has to be studied as part of a wider set of observations, the cluster of counteranxiety, counterresistance, countertransference. No less than the patient's cluster, it is now clear that the psychoanalyst's as well requires and deserves intensive study in each long-term process of therapy. How intensive it is and can be, finally, depends on the self, persona, and psyche of the coparticipants in each particular experiential field of therapy.

The Study of Shared Experience

Fundamental to the psychoanalytic study of shared experience in this field approach to direct observation of transference, resistance, anxiety and counteranxiety, counterresistance, countertransference. Implicit in the gradual movement toward this new model, yet equally important, has been a parting of the definition of these six terms from commitments to metapsychology. The first move in this direction was made when id therapists found themselves in the awkward situation of not usually being able to uncover original childhood trauma in each particular case. They started to find, instead, that they could not establish a direct correlation between the results of genetic inquiry and the objectives of current experience. As a result, their practice of psychoanalysis was increasingly threatened with becoming a psychology of pseudo-events in accordance with the metapsychologist's ability to select appropriate childhood fantasies and treat them as though they were also actual events. In order to work well, of course, it had to be accompanied by a patient's ability to find and document this metapsychology in his unconscious mind. Pseudo-events imperceptibly had to acquire the character of real events because, without their interpretive function, the whole exercise in genetic inquiry lost its logical meaning and therapeutic purpose.

The second move in this direction was made when ego-interpersonal therapists found themselves in the awkward situation of not usually being able to determine the proper expectation for relating self to society or the proper adaptation of social self to present and future cultural values in each particular case. They started to find, instead, that they could not establish a direct correlation between the adaptive point of view and cultural and interpersonal alternatives of behavior. As a result, their practice of psychoanalysis was increasingly threatened with becoming a psychology of making adjustments to vague standards of value on the basis of limited information. In order to work well, of course, it had to be supported by a patient's ability to see himself as adjustable member of the culture at large as both he and his psychoanalyst thought it really was and was really going to be;

for they had to project ego-interpersonal bridges between the rather vague standards and what they could best judge as the patient's best interests. Such ego-interpersonal bridges inevitably acquired the character of social and cultural fictions because, without personal judgment of their psychological value, the whole exercise got lost in the search for external adaptive authority whose agency and power were largely diffuse and invisible.

In working with both these models, however, it proved necessary to move toward the psychoanalytic study of shared experience on clinical grounds above all. Consider them in the following outline. First, the id therapist: he had an overweening interest in the genetic postulate. But he was impeded by three hard clinical observations. Patients ordinarily were not sexually assaulted in childhood; as a general rule, they did not even report self-induced fantasies of parental assaults either; if, after long and careful genetic inquiry, a patient finally made good the libido theory with appropriate sexual history, when he brought this interpreted history into his living present, he somehow was not capable of using this new knowledge for purposes of psychological change. Second, the ego-interpersonal therapist: he had an overweening interest in adaptation of the individual to the expectable social and cultural environment. But he, too, was hampered by other equally obstructive clinical observations. Patients did not ordinarily try to use the ego or interpersonal self to deal with social and cultural problems; when they acquired any attitude or pattern as ego-interpersonal and social adaptation, it could easily function as psychoanalyzed facade overlying a deep and untouched psychopathology, and there was no systematic way to tell it from the real thing; from the 1930's to the 1960's, strangely enough, ego-interpersonal metapsychologies became increasingly removed from the realities of the very social, cultural, and ego-interpersonal environment in which they originally claimed superiority to the id model. Not unlike undefined impulses of the biological substrate, it is clear that the culture at large is far more open and pluralistic—and far more ambiguous and multivalent, as well—than even the ego-interpersonal therapist ever thought and taught. For when patients could not be sure of which adaptations to make in their own best interests, especially in work and in love, and were too irrationally dependent on their psychoanalysts to assume the risks and responsibilities for the direction of their lives, they also did not seem readily able to accept oversimplified adaptive statements of what they ought adjust to on their psychoanalysts' say-so. And in neither the id nor the ego-interpersonal model was any clear effort made to demarcate the structure of science concerned with truth, especially that of psychoanalytic psychology, and relate it to social patterns of prudence, negotiation and compromise concerned with achieving individual best interests.

It does not follow, of course, that turning to the study of his shared experience with his patient enables the psychoanalyst, today, to solve the problems of id and ego-interpersonal therapy any better. He is no better able, in fact, to discover the secret of selecting just the right genetic or adaptive material for each particular patient; and as a result, these problems remain unsolved. Why, then, has this new psychoanalytic model of therapy been brought into being? The answer to this question can only be: because of the essential validity of the psychoanalytic enterprise as subject matter and structure of inquiry. I suppose the history of psychoanalysis could be rewritten from the point of view of these unsolved and, in our current knowledge, insoluble problems. The day they are solved, however, the earlier models may then be practiced again with new vigor and confidence; but that day is not near at hand. In response to this situation, the psychoanalytic study of shared experience represents a new attempt to take the significant and useful theoretical construct of unconscious experience, as well as a productive and workable psychological procedure, out of established metapsychologies deriving from unrealizable assumptions and pointing to dead end values that threaten continued efforts at the inquiry itself. And this third psychoanalytic model, extending and enlarging the models of id impulse and ego-interpersonal relation, represents a new attempt to put both theory and procedure on a solid footing—theory governing structure of inquiry, procedure experience of therapy. By focusing largely on the actual emergent processes and patterns, by considering afresh their genesis and function, structure and dynamism, immediacy and reflection as shared experience, by closely following the convergence of transference, resistance, anxiety and counteranxiety, counterresistance, countertransference—to learn where the shared inquiry yields clarifying information and where it bogs down in interlocking distortion – if psychoanalyst and patient succeed in working toward reconstructing the distorted self, they will then be far less concerned about the patient's fantasied childhood sexual trauma or about actual adaptation to his current expectable environment. I am not at all convinced that today's patient is very well adapted, in any event, to these particulars of biosocial and ego-interpersonal Darwinism or that he would, uncouched and untutored, naturally select them.

The New Structure of Inquiry

In 1954, I described certain procedural difficulties with both the id impulse and the ego-interpersonal models,[2] although I had not yet thought of differentiating these models in this way. At that time, I traced these difficulties in terms of Freud's stated use of the genetic postulate and Horney's stated use of the functional postulate, when each one is applied without the supplementary enrichment of the other. The only corrective to the defects of such one-sided approaches is, I still believe today, a genetic-functional approach that does not preconceive both meaning and source of the patient's trouble in advance of actual inquiry—whether it is instinctual and long-forgotten, buried in the repressed past, or cultural and ego-interpersonal, buried in current conflicts among neurotic trends, or psychological and located somewhere else again. Close description of the actual trouble becomes itself, rather, a matter of prolonged intensive inquiry, moving back and forth across past and present, applying a range of postulates beyond those of genesis and function, such as structure and dynamism, immediacy and reflection, and doing all this without preestablished perspectives on metapsychology.

But the important point is, with neither the genetic nor the functional postulate predominant, it is not necessary to attempt definition of the patient's basic problems at the very outset—even prior, in fact, to actual therapeutic inquiry—because it is now clear that his private and particular problems are not yet known and therefore cannot be resolved until much later, perhaps at terminal phases of the work. All that can be defined with any sense of adequacy, at the outset, are his presented symptoms that legitimate for him and rationalize for influential others in his life the difficult and even painful undertaking of intensive psychoanalytic inquiry over a long period of time; for psychological growing pains are not especially enjoyable, not in the conventional sense, certainly, of having a pleasant experience.

Consider the current fate of symptom perception from this point of view. With the gradual decline of interest in symptoms, since they are not basic psychological problems, the magical promise of psychoanalytic inquiry has correspondingly declined. The dependence of psychoanalysis on the medical model has proved illogical, impractical, irrational. Yet this original dependence may best account for the early prominence of the whole symptom industry. Perhaps in order to open up and explore this new field of inquiry freely, psychoanalysts first had to mask interest in the human psyche behind medical therapy of nervous symptoms so that they could then formulate psychic function as somatic tautology. In doing this since the turn of the century, they have produced a most exciting and informative chapter–so far unwritten–in the recent history of the human sciences. For this movement away from models of id impulse and ego-interpersonal relation toward that of shared experience is fundamentally a movement away from the medical model of all psychoanalytic therapies. Actually, taking off the mask of somatic symptoms reveals a dynamic field of psychology that is valid in its own terms and workable under its own conditions. In a certain obvious metaphorical sense, it signifies removal of the symptom of self-doubt from the body of psychoanalytic knowledge.

Instead of id therapy's largely genetic study of real or imagined childhood sexual trauma, and instead of ego-interpersonal therapy's largely functional study of adaptation to the expectable environment, a new approach is under way. Psychoanalysts are now looking more and more intently into the shared experience of the psychoanalytic field of inquiry itself for significant definable observations of transference, resistance, anxiety. And they are also looking to immediate contexts of that same shared experience for their limits and possibilities of exploration as set by significant definable observations of counteranxiety, counterresistance, countertransference. This new interest in shared qualities of the psychoanalytic experience, insofar as they are available for study under actual psychoanalytic inquiry, is essentially a psychological interest that may eventually encompass any process or pattern of human psyche. What does human psyche mean in this connection? It is that field of processes and patterns the relation of whose conscious and unconscious aspects are the concern of psychoanalysts, who are now trying harder to do what the name of their discipline says they do, and they are trying to do it with as little obfuscation as possible. In a word: to psychoanalyze the psyche. And what of this new interest in shared qualities of psychoanalytic experience? It represents the surrender of false metapsychological certainties in favor of the risks and responsibilities of reliable psychological knowledge, to the extent that self-knowledge is available in psychoanalytic inquiry. This is not to write off metapsychology as meaningless or even superfluous, or to write it out of the enduring concerns of psychoanalysis but, rather and as changing emphasis, to shift the focus of inquiry away from value systems over into empirical and systematic knowledge, from speculative philosophy to philosophy of science, from interpretive metapsychology to psychological inquiry.

With this major shift in emphasis, placing the order of metapsychology on a working basis of open and radical pluralism, psychoanalysts holding different value systems should be able to work together in what they commonly describe as the same psychological field of inquiry. And of equal importance, too, particular psychoanalysts and particular patients who must in some way differ over some aspect of value systems should also be able to work together in what they commonly describe as the same experiential field of therapy. The objective of this major shift is to make way for a new psychoanalytic structure that is not committed to any one of the many metapsychologies now in use–biological, sociological, psychological–and does not require creation of still another new structure every time some psychoanalyst gets a bright idea about human values and beliefs, or sees a new slant on the philosophy of psychological problems and their resolu-

TABLE 1

SYMBOLS OF REPRESENTATION

Orders of Psychoanalytic Inquiry				
Empirical		Systematic		Interpretive
Observation	Definition	Postulation	Theory	Metapsychology
(1)	(2)	(3)	(4)	(5)
transference t_n	transference t	genesis G	unconscious experience U	Freudian [M_1]
resistance r_n	resistance r	function F		Adlerian [M_2]
anxiety a_n	anxiety a	structure S		Jungian [M_3]
counter-anxiety ca_n	counter-anxiety ca	dynamism D		Rankian [M_4]
counter-resistance cr_n	counter-resistance cr	immediacy I		• • •
counter-transference ct_n	counter-transference ct	reflection R		• • • [M_n]

tions. For the integration of all such new value systems, such as, even, the model of shared experience, which I happen to value highly, does not cause any logical or scientific difficulties if the overall structure of psychoanalytic knowledge rests on empirical and systematic foundations, to which a variety of interpretive capstones may be added. TABLE 1 depicts their arrangement and symbolization.[3] (See also References 4–7). By making the order of metapsychology open and pluralistic, then, psychoanalysts no longer have to create whole new systems of psychoanalysis whenever they introduce new value systems at the fifth order of metapsychology or, empirically, make new observations at the first order and define them as the second or, systematically, construct new postulates and theory at the third and fourth orders.

To summarize this significance of the new psychoanalytic structure: aspects of its various orders may change in the future, and probably will, as the result of making new observation, definition, postulation and theory, or extending and enlarging any such constituents already established in the structure. But the general map of its empirical and systematic foundations is firm and secure. It is no longer either necessary or possible for any single psychoanalyst, at present, to create the whole structure afresh in outline or anew in terminology whenever he makes a new and important contribution to its order of interpretive metapsychology.

It is possible to take this view, at the present time, because it is possible to outline and apply a psychoanalytic structure that receives various systems of value that parallel and even counter those already established in the history of this discipline by Freud, Adler, Jung, Rank and others. In this respect, the new psychoanalytic structure is in accord with the democratic ideal of every man being finally responsible for the place he takes and activities he undertakes in his ego-interpersonal environment–which holds true for all psychoanalytic patients, of course, in or outside the experiential field of therapy. Otherwise, psychoanalytic therapists become social agents of adjustment and adaptation to the social order as it is. And if disturbed exponents of our present and dissenting culture find it practically impossible, on account of this, to avail themselves of the healing resources of psychoanalysis, there is no doubt they are right.

References

1. WOLSTEIN, B. 1967. Theory of Psychoanalytic Therapy : 24–37. Grune & Stratton. New York.
2. WOLSTEIN, B. 1954. Transference. 1964. Second Edit. : 83–199. Grune & Stratton. New York.
3. WOLSTEIN, B. 1967. Theory of Psychoanalytic Therapy : 157. Grune & Stratton. New York.
4. WOLSTEIN, B. 1965. Notes on Psychoanalytic Structure. *In* Selected Papers on Psychotherapy. L. Kingsley *et al.*, Eds. : 3–31. Adelphi University. Garden City, L. I.
5. WOLSTEIN, B. 1968. Determination and freedom in psychoanalysis. Amer. J. Psychoanal. **28**: 65–68.
6. WOLSTEIN, B. 1969. Concerning feminine mystique and masculine myth. *In* Modern Woman. G. Goldman and D. Milman, Eds. : 97–101. Charles C Thomas. Springfield, Ill.
7. WOLSTEIN, B. 1969. The new psychoanalytic structure. Amer. J. Psychother. **23**: 260–270.

Discussion

DR. SAMUEL A. WEISS (*Yeshiva University*): A number of questions occurred to me while listening to your paper, Dr. Wolstein. First, it seems remarkable that you dealt with the id and ego, while the superego was absent from the discussion. You say that patients appear to suffer far less from unsatisfied biological needs and failed social securities than from blocked striving for psychic freedom and personal fulfillment. Perhaps what they miss most in life is a sense of "meaning" which might be related to the satisfaction of superego needs. Many existentialists have been saturating us so thoroughly with the supposed meaninglessness of existence that the antiplacebo "life is absurd" is now in vogue like the maxi-dress. It covers everything but makes it uninteresting as well. Perhaps the eviction of positive aspects of the superego from the consideration of some analysts and therapists is responsible for the feelings of meaninglessness and purposelessness in life even while more id and ego need are satisfied. Perhaps that is why even the much vaunted group psychotherapies have been failing (as mentioned by another listener) and are now being converted by some into group orgies of sense satisfaction? In any case, the total omission of the superego from your talk made me wonder. Second, your statement as regards the supposed reduction of interest in symptoms, on the part of patients, is surprising. The main factor driving a patient to contact us has been precisely symptoms, harbinges of suffering. It is the symptoms and suffering that propel the client into treatment. Of course, once he learns the rules of the psychoanalytic game, he can perhaps be seduced into ignoring them temporarily while one psychological-archeological layer after another is uncovered. Unless, however, the symptoms are ultimately dealt with, and eliminated or subdued, the patient will leave in midstream. In fact, the new behavior therapists proclaim that there is no psychological problem but the symptom and that they are its prophets! Third, your approach of abandoning *content* and concentrating mainly on the interactional *process* seems to be a complete reaction formation against dealing with crucial symptoms, whether directly, as the behavior therapists claim they do, or indirectly, as other psychotherapists and analysts do. A patient may leave us once he is symptomatically happier or, if he is wiser, more motivated and economically able, he may realize that deeper conflicts exist within him which should be explored. Or, if he has no such realization, other symptoms, originally flattened by the pressure of the now dissipated presenting symptom, may expand and bid both patient and therapist to take notice. Symptoms may be second-class citizens to us, the analysts and therapists, but they are certainly first-class ego-aliens to our deeply suffering patient. It seems to me that you have given short shrift to two important problems in treatment- 1) symptoms and 2) giving the patient, or helping him discover, real meaning in life.

DR. WOLSTEIN: I wish Dr. Weiss had brought his couch, you know, and I'd get my defense mechanism analyzed. You asked many questions and some of them extend beyond the range of my paper. I don't ignore the superego, and I don't think anybody in the history of psychoanalysis does, but what I've done in selecting my terminology is to use what I call Freud's first model of therapy, id therapy, because essentially the guiding principle of interpretation in the general introductory lectures was the libido theory, which was essentially an id therapy. You may remember that in the new introductory lectures, which Freud published in 1933, I think, he said that he was developing new theories of metapsychology that included the id ego-superego distinction. However, he never really changed his basic psychoanalytic procedure, that is, his basic design of therapy. So I think it's fair to say that Freud's first major design for psychoanalytic therapy was an id therapy. Now the second model of therapy I call an ego-interpersonal model, because I think that people like Sullivan and Hartmann are working with the same clinical material, and I think they are working in different frames of reference, and in different terminology, or in different metapsychologies. But I don't think that it would be fair to either Reich, or Anna Freud, or Hartmann, or Sullivan, or Horney, or any of the people who work in this second model of therapy to call that a superego model, because it essentially is not. It's an attempt to work with the autonomous directive functions of the ego, or the interpersonal self.

There has been too much superego. It's not that there has been insufficient interpretation of the values, but *too much* interpretation of the values. And psychoanalysis came to be known as a kind of, you know, an adjustment therapy, a therapy of how to make it. For example, if you weren't doing well on your job, or if you were having troubles with your marriage, well in an id therapy model, of course, the major kinds of symptoms all revolved around sexual functioning. The thing to do was see an analyst and he'd straighten you out, as though you were some kind of mechanical object. And that's the thing I think the model of shared experience is trying to eliminate; we try to get away from the idea that a person is that kind of mechanical thing, that when he brings in a symptom, it's not simply a question of some behavioral disorder that he has. And we're not trying to change his "spark plugs" so his "car" goes better. There's something the matter in the psyche of the individual, and the purpose of psychoanalysis is to conduct an exploration of this psyche. These are just rough comments to questions that would require a whole paper.

DR. SELIG (*Low Cost Therapy Plan, N. J.*): We have so much to do with the prevalence of disturbance that we need to function in groups, so I am trying to understand your use of the phrase, "shared experience" as a group phenomenon. I don't know if I'm correct in this, but I heard no reference to the use of groups. We are also coming to the end of the road in the use of groups and we're having the same kinds of a failures even in shared experiences, if I may try to combine the two. Where do we go from here? This brings to mind Franz Alexander's paper, I believe in the Journal of International Psychiatry, in which he really threw a curve and said that so far as he was concerned, all psychoanalytic phenomenon theory could be reduced to learning theory in the long run. Would you have any comments on this?

DR. WOLSTEIN: I think I'd better give Dr. Weiss back his couch and get my defense mechanisms out. I didn't refer to groups because I think that group therapy is an outgrowth of ego-interpersonal therapy, which deals essentially with social communication, or adaptation of the individual to the group. The model of shared experience is concerned essentially with the person's relationship to himself, and how he relates *to* his relationships to the group. I think that the reason why group therapy is phasing out is the same reason why symptom therapy is phasing out. I think it has to do with the fact that there's ostensibly something new going on in the culture, and I feel that something new *is* going on. It has to do with people's more intensive interest in what's going on inside themselves, or their inner perception, and I don't mean to line myself up here with the people who are in the counter-culture. But if you look around at the new interests, mysticisms and the occult, extrasensory perception, even astrology, and so on, I think that all of these interests, if you don't take them literally, but as symptoms, suggest the fact that people are not satisfied with the established rationalistic categories of experience. And the problem with group therapy is that it has become and has been used essentially as an adaptive therapeutic technique rather than, and I guess this would be the basic distinction I'm trying to make, an exploratory technique, a psychological exploration. Now, I have not called this new form of therapy "shared experience" in order to get involved in some derivative social, or socialistic type of thing here. My main interest in calling it shared experience is to emphasize the fact that both the psychoanalyst and the patient are involved in a joint inquiry, that is, to distinguish the relationship between psychoanalyst and the patient today from, say, the relationship that existed in the classical freudian position. Some of you may have heard about, or may have read a new book called Brother Animal, in which Victor Tausk is supposed to have committed suicide over the fact that he couldn't get analyzed. He was obviously disturbed, but he had a basic difference of opinion with Freud as to the kind of model of therapy or the kind of relationship he was supposed to have with a patient. Freud insisted that the analyst remain the mirror, and wouldn't even take Tausk. I don't want to get involved in the whole story, but I recommend the book just to get an idea of how geniuses really work, and how they manage to establish their reputations. But, the important point I'm trying to get at with shared experience is the fact that the analyst and the patient are involved in a common field of experience, a joint inquiry, and that the analyst's personality, psyche, distortions and anxiety, defense mechanisms and resistances, and transference from his past, are all involved in this field of experience, and, at appropriate times, may even become parts of the inquiry. Thus, the shared experience model has to do not so much with the matter of groups, but rather reflects especially on the relationship of the psychoanalyst to his patient, the former becoming a part of the inquiry rather than remaining a mirror, or as Franz Alexander used to describe the analyst, a therapeutic expert who is basically uninvolved. We're willing to try and become involved and we're willing to try to take the psychoanalytic method as far as we can take it.

MRS. SCHALLER (*Bowling Green State University, Ohio*): I'm an educator, so I listen with a layman's ears. But I wondered if you saw patients after traumatic events, after symptoms are very pronounced? I would like to know if you have any suggestions for educators that could help these patients. We see children when they're young, when maybe the nucleus of these symptoms is there, and I wondered if for educators there were any suggestions that would influence our approaches to children? This may be tangential to what you are talking about, but may I have your views anyway?

DR. WOLSTEIN: I'm glad that you raised this question because it gives me an opportunity to emphasize a point that I was trying to make in the paper. And that is, in the new psychoanalytic structure there is no one metapsychology; because of this I think that the question whether psychoanalysts have suggestions for education or for politics is significant. In the last election, or was it two elections ago, psychoanalysts became involved in the psychoanalysis of a candidate and an editor of a journal was sued. I think that it's about time that psychoanalysts stopped playing the role of priests, that is, secular priests in the culture, and really tended to the business that their name says they are involved in, which is, the psychoanalysis of the psyche. If psychoanalysts later specialize in education, and they offer suggestions on how children should be educated, I think that they would be speaking rather as educators than as psychoanalysts. And I would say the same holds true for psychoanalysts who are trying to become involved in any other field.

I think that the attitude that psychoanalysists have a metapsychology they can preach to the world is one of the problems that we are still suffering from, starting with the period of id therapy when Freud was trying to work out a metapsychology or philosophy of experience that was supposed to stretch out into all domains. Psychologists were even supposed to explain why the Trobrianders didn't have the same family relationship that people in Vienna had. And when Malinowski tried to demonstrate this, then Jones said that it had to do with the sexual ignorance of savages. What I'm driving at is that the classical psychoanalytic view attempted a universalistic conception in the tradition of 18th- to 19th-century German philosophy. And psychoanalysts today, especially those trained in this country since the war, have narrowed down their interests quite a bit and are willing to proceed with psychoanalytic exploration as best they can, and leave education to the educators.

PERCEPTUAL FUNCTIONING IN SCHIZOPHRENIA: IMPLICATIONS FOR THE STUDY OF PERCEPTUAL PROCESSES

Irving B. Weiner, Ph.D.
University of Rochester School of Medicine and Dentistry
Rochester, N. Y.

Some 20 years ago Norman Cameron[13] presented an important paper on behavior pathology as part of a symposium on perceptual organization. He commented then that the inclusion of his topic in a symposium on perception was noteworthy, and he justified its inclusion by stressing the "principle of continuity," namely, that all of the attitudes and responses found in behavior pathology are related to, or derived from, aspects of normal behavior. Partly as a long-range consequence of that symposium, which was published under the title Perception: An Approach to Personality, it is hardly necessary now to defend or encourage perceptual approaches to the study of abnormal behavior.

It is still relevant, however, to stress that the results of such studies have implications for perceptual functioning in general and for normal as well as abnormal personality variations. This paper will illustrate the broad implications of perceptual studies of abnormal behavior through a brief review of what has been demonstrated about perceptual functioning in schizophrenia.

Basic Notions

The basic notions of perceptual functioning in schizophrenia were set down by Eugen Bleuler[5] in his classic 1911 monograph. According to Bleuler, schizophrenia does not entail any primary impairment of the capacity for perception, and any apparent exception to this fact can always be traced to disturbances of attention or cognition (see pp. 57–58). On the other hand, Bleuler continues, the schizophrenic person's perceptions of himself and his environment are secondarily distorted by *autism*; autism, which Bleuler posits as a primary feature of schizophrenia, implies that perceptions are determined more by internal needs than by external reality. In elaborating the concept of autism, Bleuler implicitly endorsed the principle of continuity mentioned by Cameron. He stressed that all people demonstrate needs to seek substitutes in fantasy for unsatisfactory realities, but that the schizophrenic is extreme in the extent to which he brings his perceptual experience into harmony with his emotional needs, even at the expense of shutting off almost the entire reality of perceptual stimulation (pp. 63–68, 373–374).

The past 50 years, and especially the last 20, have seen enormous advances in the sophistication of theory construction and research strategies in the study of perceptual processes[30,77] and of schizophrenia.[51,59,67] Yet for the most part this impressive volume of work has not substantially challenged Bleuler's formulation of perceptual functioning in schizophrenia.

With regard to perceptual processes, the "new look" that emerged in the late 1940's and early 1950's provided empirical confirmation of the notions of need-influenced perception and perceptual defense on which the concept of autism is based. The landmark studies of impoverished children who overestimated the size of coins[7] and of adults who avoided conscious perception of tachisticopically presented taboo words[20,50] quantified normal manifestations of the same autistic process that in more extreme form produces schizophrenic distortions of perceptual reality.

As for schizophrenia, research data have supported the observations of Bleuler and other clinicians[2,10,22,44,84] that schizophrenics are more likely than other people to misperceive their environment and themselves, and furthermore, that they become increasingly prone to such perceptual distortions in the face of personally relevant, threatening, or otherwise affectively charged stimuli. Schizophrenic subjects give a significantly higher percentage of inaccurate form percepts in their response to the Rorschach test than do either normal or neurotic subjects, and poor form perception is considered the single most reliable psychodiagnostic indicator of schizophrenia (see Reference 85, pp. 109–110). In the auditory sphere, Moon and colleagues[54] report that schizophrenics make significantly more errors than do normals when they are asked simply to repeat words spoken to them one at a time. Since Moon's group scored errors only when the word repeated was neither an acceptable association to the stimulus word nor phonetically similar to it, the relatively inaccurate performances of the schizophrenics appeared attributable to their mishearing the words more frequently than did the normal subjects.

Other work has illustrated the tendency of schizophrenics to misperceive people in their environment. Iscoe and Veldman[36] found that schizophrenics made significantly more errors than normal subjects in arranging pictures of faces according to the amount of happiness the faces expressed. Other studies have also indicated that schizophrenics are less able than normals to provide accurate descriptions of people they have met or whose autobiographies they have read[34,37] and less able to discriminate accurately between the typical attitudes and roles of men, women, and children.[52,53]

With respect to their perception of themselves, there is considerable evidence that schizophrenics differ both from normal controls and from psychologically disturbed but nonschizophrenic subjects in their capacity to estimate the size of their own body parts. When asked to compare the size of their own hands, feet, and other body parts with photographs of them, schizophrenics have been found either to underestimate or overestimate their actual size.[8,15,16,82] Schizophrenics are also less able than normal subjects to recognize photographs of their own bodies,[3] and both male and female schizophrenics report a larger number of distorted body experiences than do normal men and women, including such experiences as small body size, loss of body boundary, blocking of body openings, and perception of the body as dirty.[21,23] Finally there is evidence that male schizophrenics are significantly more likely than normal men to report hallucinatory experiences regarding their genitals and delusions of being women or no longer men,[29] and that female schizophrenics significantly more often than normal women experience genital hallucinosis, delusions of change of size or shape of their genitalia, and delusions of changing sex.[28]

Studies of perceptual recognition and discrimination and of size estimates have also confirmed that the relative inaccuracy of schizophrenic subjects tends to increase in the presence of personally relevant or affectively charged stimuli. In recognizing and discriminating between pictures, schizophrenics to a greater extent than normals make more perceptual errors with pictures weighted with human content than with those devoid of it,[18] more on pictures with sexual than nonsexual content,[1] and more on pictures of scenes intended to depict positive or negative affective interactions than on pictures of neutral scenes.[19,75] As for size estimates, schizophrenics, but not normal controls, have been observed to misjudge the sizes of pictures of psychiatric patients but not of psychiatric aides,[56] to overestimate the typical circumferences of a scoop of ice cream and a cigar, but not that of a button,[58] and to judge correctly the size of a baseball while overestimating the size of their body parts.[15,16]

COMPLICATING LINES OF RESEARCH

Although these and other empirical data support Bleuler's formulation, three other lines of research complicate our current understanding of perceptual functioning in schizophrenia: first, several aspects of perceptual disturbance traditionally associated with schizophrenia have proved neither universal among schizophrenics nor exclusive to the schizophrenic condition; second, numerous studies of perceptual functioning in which attempts were made to remove all contextual and affective meaning from the stimuli, that is, maximization of the so-called "autochthonous" factors in perception, have still yielded significant differences between schizophrenic and normal subjects; and third, considerable data indicate that many of the influences of personality on perception are mediated by attentional variables and cognitive dispositions that cut across diagnostic lines.

Heterogeneity

Recent research in schizophrenia is marked by increasing recognition of the heterogeneity of the disorder along a wide range of personality dimensions,[45,67] including the non-universality of perceptual disturbance in schizophrenia. In a study of size estimates of pictures with thematic content, for example, Harris[32] found no differences between the mean size estimates of normal and schizophrenic groups; however, the schizophrenic group was considerably more variable than the normals, and when Harris divided them into subsamples of good-premorbid and poor-premorbid schizophrenics, he learned that the good-premorbids had significantly underestimated the size of the pictures relative to the normals, whereas the poor-premorbids had significantly overestimated picture size. In a similar study, unfortunately with a different outcome, Zahn[90] observed overestimation of picture size by good-premorbid schizophrenic subjects relative to normals but no differences between normals and poor-premorbids.

In other relevant work acutely disturbed schizophrenics have been found to demonstrate greater perceptual closure than normals, and chronic schizophrenics, less tendency to closure than normals;[72,73] reactive schizophrenics have shown significantly less difficulty than process schizophrenics in perceiving and integrating auditory stimuli;[35] and acute schizophrenics have generally proved less inaccurate in their form perception on the Rorschach than have chronic schizophrenics (Reference 85, pp. 244–245).

Johannsen[38,39] has reviewed these and other data that appear to indicate decreasing performance with chronicity on a variety of perceptual tasks. He suggests the possibility of a widespread perceptual deficit in schizophrenia that becomes apparent only after a long duration of the disturbance, and he proposes the following framework to account for available data: (a) in responding to complex, affectively charged perceptual stimuli, acute schizophrenics will perform less well than normal subjects, and chronic schizophrenics will demonstrate even greater deficits than acute schizophrenics; (b) when elements of complexity and affectivity are minimized on perceptual tasks, acute schizophrenics will perform similarly to normal subjects; but (c) with increasing chronicity, schizophrenics will demonstrate increasingly marked deficits involving increasing numbers of perceptual functions.

Distinctions between paranoid and nonparanoid schizophrenics also figure prominently in evaluating perceptual deficit. For example, paranoid schizophrenics have been observed not to differ significantly from normal subjects in their perception of apparent movement, whereas nonparanoid schizophrenics demonstrate a noticeable deficit in perception of optimal apparent movement.[62] Paranoid schizophrenics are also less likely than nonparanoid subjects to demonstrate grossly inaccurate form perception on the Rorschach (Reference 85, p. 313).

Silverman recently pointed out that, in general, groups of poor-premorbid, long-term hospitalized, and nonparanoid schizophrenics have behaved similarly on various psychological measures and differently from groups of good-premorbid, early-term hospitalized, and paranoid schizophrenic subjects (Reference 71, pp. 226–227):

> The former groups, clinically more withdrawn, evidencing more thought disorder, and apparently more preoccupied, have demonstrated reduced perceptual responsiveness on a variety of laboratory procedures. . . . The latter groups typically have evidenced normal or extraordinary perceptual response to stimulation. . . . In a number of perceptual studies the performance scores of the two kinds of schizophrenic groups actually have deviated in opposite directions from those of nonclinical comparison groups.

Nonexclusiveness

In addition to demonstrating such heterogeneity in perceptual functioning among schizophrenic subgroups, clinical and research findings have indicated that many perceptual disturbances traditionally associated with schizophrenia occur in nonschizophrenic people as well. Tucker and coworkers,[74] for example, asked different clinical groups about their personal experience with several subjective perceptions traditionally associated with schizophrenia, such as "noises all seem to be louder." They found no significant differences among schizophrenic, depressed, character-disordered, and organic patient groups in either the mean number of distorted perceptual experiences they reported or the percent of each diagnostic group reporting them. In the studies of body experience by Fisher and Seidner,[21,23] similarly, neurotic as well as schizophrenic subjects reported significantly more distorted body experiences than did normals.

Hallucinatory phenomena that occur independently of any drug or other artificially imposed hallucinogenic influence (e.g. sensory deprivation, sleep deprivation) are often a major clue to schizophrenic disorder, yet hallucinatory experiences are also observed in brain-damaged, neurotic, and even normal persons.[4,24,46,63] Frieske and Wilson[25] have recently reported an impressive similarity in the formal perceptual qualities of visual hallucinations experienced among groups of schizophrenic, organic, and affectively psychotic patients. Poor perceptual accuracy on the Rorschach has been noted among brain-damaged and mentally retarded as well as schizophrenic subjects, and psychodiagnostic indices of inaccurate perception imply schizophrenic impairment only when such other conditions can be ruled out (Reference 85, pp. 110–112).

Autochthonous factors

Studies maximizing autochthonous factors in perception have, for the most part, utilized simple geometric figures as the perceptual stimuli. Thus schizophrenics have been found to be less accurate than normal subjects in simply judging the length of lines, a task in which cognitive complexity and personal or affective relevance are presumably at a minimum.[14,17] Geometric figures and abstract images have also been employed to study perceptual constancy in schizophrenics. In this work schizophrenic subjects have demonstrated significantly less distance constancy than normals, shown both with binocular and monocular perception;[42,81,83] they have displayed significantly less shape constancy than normal and patient controls;[79] and they have been found in some instances to demonstrate less size constancy than normal and neurotic subjects[31,47,78] and, in other instances, more size constancy than normals and neurotics.[33,57,61] Other studies have also found significantly smaller figural aftereffects in schizophrenic than in normal subjects.[40,41,86,87]

These studies merit closer critical scrutiny than is possible within the limits of this paper, with respect both to research design and, in the case of size constancy, the contrary findings. For present purposes it is sufficient merely to grant that such data raise the possibility of a basic perceptual deficit in schizophrenia that, contrary to Bleulerian notions, cannot be attributed to threatening contextual aspects of the stimuli. Yet it is important to recall Bleuler's comment that any apparent exceptions to the schizophrenic's basic perceptual intactness can always be traced to disturbances of attention or cognition. In this comment Bleuler anticipated by many years a number of current theoretical interpretations of performance deficit in schizophrenia in which perceptual disturbances, no matter how apparently primary, are attributed to more basic disorders of attention and information processing.

Attention Variables

A number of independently conceived notions of schizophrenic deficit, each derived from a body of research data, have in recent years combined to suggest that observed cognitive deficits in schizophrenia derive essentially from the schizophrenic's inability to establish and maintain an adaptive and appropriate focus of attention on relevant aspects of his experience. Thus Shakow[64,65] concludes from his extensive laboratory studies that schizophrenics are deficient in their capacity to maintain segmental set, that is, to prevent extraneous stimuli from disrupting their focus of attention. McGhie[48] reviews other findings that appear to demonstrate a marked disorder of selective attention in schizophrenics, and he notes that the relative inability of schizophrenic subjects to screen out irrelevant, extraneous information has a particularly detrimental effect in situations that demand accurate perception and recall of information. Weckowicz and Blewett[80] also attribute abnormalities of perception in schizophrenia to an inability to attend selectively or select relevant information.

Other researchers have used different language to describe the same phenomenon. Payne[55] reviews data that led him to posit "overinclusiveness" as a basic aspect of cognitive deficit in schizophrenia. Following the earlier ideas of Cameron,[11,12] Payne uses "overinclusiveness" to describe an incapacity to filter out the relevant information in a stimulus field. Venables[76] infers from his experimental work that schizophrenics suffer an "input dysfunction" characterized primarily by a broadened level of attention and a cognitively disruptive sensory overload.

Reviews of the research literature on schizophrenia[6,9,45] indicate that this type of interference theory, that is, the notion of some interference with the capacity to establish and maintain a relevant focus of attention, is probably more powerful in accounting for available data than any of the other extant theoretical interpretations of observed cognitive deficit in schizophrenia. Thus it may be that any apparently primary perceptual abnormality in schizophrenia, whether in size estimation, constancy, closure, or whatever, derives secondarily from a basic impairment of the capacity to attend to and process stimulus information.

Disordered attention, however, like disordered perception, is neither universal nor consistently demonstrable among schizophrenics. Even within a sample of chronic schizophrenics, the ability to maintain set varies widely in relation to the individual patient's degree of disorganization.[60] Shakow,[64,65] furthermore, reports that hebephrenic schizophrenics display particular inability to maintain a segmental set, whereas paranoid schizophrenics hold even more firmly and narrowly than do normal subjects to an established set. McGhie[49] similarly indicates that in his studies hebphrenic subjects were notably distractible, whereas paranoid subjects had even less difficulty than normal controls in fixating attention on one of a number of competing stimuli.

Cognitive Dispositions

It is next relevant to turn to the implications of cognitive dispositions for the understanding of perceptual functioning in schizophrenia. The work of George Klein and Riley Gardner and their collaborators over a number of years[26,27,43] has demonstrated that various polarized perceptual attitudes (e.g. leveling versus sharpening of differences, tolerance versus resistance to the unstable, constriction versus flexibility) become characterological traits, that is, essential aspects of personality organization that are relatively persistent and enduring in the face of intercurrent influences.

Two such cognitive dispositions that have been studied in relation to schizophrenia are field independence-dependence and scanning control-field articulation, both of which significantly influence many aspects of perceptual functioning.[26,27,89] Witkin[88] reviews data that relate field independence-dependence to symptoms of psychological disorder but not to any gross nosological category; specifically, he reports that schizophrenic subjects are heterogeneous with regard to field independence-dependence, with paranoid schizophrenics tending to be field-independent and catatonic schizophrenics field-dependent.

Silverman[68,69,70] has utilized the principles of scanning control and field articulation to account for a number of aspects of cognitive functioning in subgroups of schizophrenics. He concludes from various data that paranoid schizophrenics tend to scan their perceptual environment extensively and articulate incoming information carefully, whereas nonparanoid subtypes demonstrate minimal scanning and undifferentiated field articulation. Similarly, acute schizophrenics tend to exercise relatively differentiated field articulation and chronic schizophrenics relatively undifferentiated field articulation.

To these principles, which can account for much of the data on perceptual functioning in schizophrenia, Silverman adds the important notion of "ideational gating." According to Silverman, the ideational gating mechanism filters out disturbing connotative environmental inputs and is the ultimate schizophrenic defense mechanism. This principle brings us full circle to the Bleulerian concept of autism, namely, that the internal needs of schizophrenics inordinately distort their perceptions of themselves and their environment. Like other perceptual phenomena, the gating mechanism is demonstrably more characteristic of some types of schizophrenia than others, as summarized by Silverman (Reference 71, p. 245):

> Chronic, nonparanoid, and "poor-premorbid" schizophrenic types attend more than is normal to the sensory attributes of perceptual-ideational inputs and less than is normal to connotative attributes. This is especially the case when the inputs connote psychological threat or are extremely unpleasant in their affective tone; connotative attributes of such perceptual-ideational inputs are often gated – i.e., excluded from awareness.

Implications for the Study of Perceptual Processes

This brief overview of the research on perceptual functioning in schizophrenia points up two directions of increasing sophistication in research design: one involves increasing attention to the stimuli, particularly with regard to whether they contain anxiety- or affect-arousing properties that induce apparent but only secondary perceptual dysfunctioning in schizophrenic subjects; the second involves consideration of individual differences, with regard both to differences between subgroups of schizophrenics in their capacity to attend and process information and to cognitive disposition that cut across diagnostic lines.

This consideration of individual differences has significant implications for any attempt to isolate and examine basic perceptual processes. Consistently with the principle of continuity mentioned at the beginning of this paper, it is reasonable to expect that nonschizophrenic as well as schizophrenic subjects will differ in the level and relevance of their attention. Furthermore, differences among nonschizophrenic and nonclinical as well as schizophrenic groups are readily demonstrable on field independence-dependence,[89] field scanning-articulation and ideational gating,[71] and probably a host of other cognitive dispositions, some known and others as yet unrecognized, any of which can operate as significant independent variables in studies of perceptual processes. Attempts to study basic perceptual processes, even within presumably normal subject groups, accordingly require careful assessment of the influence of attentional states and of known or perhaps unsuspected cognitive dispositions that can influence the dependent perceptual variable under investigation.

Shakow[66] has discussed at length the implications for general psychology of experimental studies of schizophrenia. As outlined in this paper, it is particularly clear that efforts to understand schizophrenic disorder have highlighted types of sample heterogeneity and individual differences that must be considered in efforts to study perceptual processes.

References

1. Arey, L. B. 1960. The indirect representation of sexual stimuli by schizophrenic and normal subjects. J. Abnorm. Soc. Psychol. **61:** 424–431.
2. Arieti, S. 1959. Schizophrenia: the manifest symptomatology, the psychodynamic and formal mechanisms. *In* American Handbook of Psychiatry. S. Arieti, Ed. : Basic Books. New York.
3. Arhhoff, F. N. & E. N. Damianopoulos. 1964. Self-body recognition and schizophrenia. J. Gen. Psychol. **70:** 353–361.
4. Baldwin, M. 1962. Hallucinations in neurological syndromes. *In* Hallucinations. L. J. West, Ed. : 77–85. Grune & Stratton. New York.
5. Bleuler, E. 1950. Dementia Praecox or the Group of Schizophrenias. International Universities Press. New York.
6. Broen, W. E. 1968. Schizophrenia: Research and Theory. Academic Press. New York.
7. Bruner, J. S. & C. C. Goodman. 1947. Value and need as organizing factors in perception. J. Abnorm. Soc. Psychol. **42:** 33–44.
8. Burton, A. & J. Adkins. 1961. Perceived size of self-image body parts in schizophrenia. Archives of General Psychiatry **5:** 131–140.
9. Buss, A. H. & P. J. Lang. 1965. Psychological deficit in schizophrenia: I. Affect, reinforcement, and concept attainment. J. Abnorm. Psychol. **70:** 2–24.
10. Bychowski, G. 1943. Disorders in the body-image in the clinical pictures of psychoses. J. Nerv. Ment. Dis. **97:** 310–334.
11. Cameron, N. 1939. Schizophrenic thinking in a problem-solving situation. J. Ment. Sci. **85:** 1012–1035.
12. Cameron, N. 1939. Deterioration and regression in schizophrenic thinking. J. Abnorm. Soc. Psychol. **34:** 265–270.

13. CAMERON, N. 1951. Perceptual organization and behavior psychology. *In* Perception: An Approach to Personality. R. R. Blake & G. V. Ramsey, Eds. : 283–306. Ronald Press. New York.
14. CHAMBERS, J. L. 1956. Perceptual judgment and associative learning ability of schizophrenics and nonpsychotics. J. Consult. Psychol. **20:** 211–214.
15. CLEVELAND, S. E. 1960. Judgments of body size in a schizophrenia and a control group. Psychol. Reports **7:** 304.
16. CLEVELAND, S. E., S. FISHER, E. E. REITMAN & P. ROTHAUS. 1962. Perception of body size in schizophrenia. Arch. Gen. Psychiat. **7:** 277–285.
17. COOPER, R. 1960. Objective measures of perception in schizophrenics and normals. J. Consult. Psychol. **24:** 209–214.
18. DAVIS, R. H. & R. W. HARRINGTON. 1957. The effect of stimulus class on the problem-solving behavior of schizophrenics and normals. J. Abnorm. Soc. Psychol. **54:** 126–128.
19. DUNN, W. L. 1954. Visual discrimination of schizophrenic subjects as a function of stimulus meaning. J. Personal. **23:** 48–64.
20. ERIKSEN, C. W. 1951. Perceptual defense as a function of unacceptable needs. J. Abnorm. Soc. Psychol. **46:** 557–564.
21. FISHER, S. 1964. Body image and psychopathology. Arch. Gen. Psychiat. **10:** 519–529.
22. FISHER, S. & S. E. CLEVELAND. 1958. Body Image and Personality. Van Nostrand. Princeton, N. J.
23. FISHER, S. & R. SEIDNER. 1963. Body experiences of schizophrenic, neurotic, and normal women. J. Nerv. Ment. Dis. **137:** 252–257.
24. FORRER, G. R. 1960. Benign auditory and visual hallucinations. Arch. Gen. Psychiat. **3:** 95–98.
25. FRIESKE, D. A. & W. P. WILSON. 1966. Formal qualities of hallucinations: A comparative study of the visual hallucinations in patients with schizophrenic, organic, and affective psychosis. In Psychopathology of Schizophrenia. P. H. Hoch & Zubin, Eds. : 49–62. Grune & Stratton. New York.
26. GARDNER, R. W., P. S. HOLZMAN, G. S. KLEIN, H. B. LINTON & D. P. SPENCE. 1959. Cognitive control: A study of individual consistencies in cognitive behavior. Psychol. Issues **1**(4).
27. GARDNER, R. W., D. N. JACKSON & S. J. MESSICK. 1960. Personality organization in cognitive controls and intellectual abilities. Psychol. Issues **2**(8).
28. GITTLESON, N. L. & K. DAWSON-BUTTERWORTH. 1967. Subjective ideas of sexual change in female schizophrenics. Brit. J. Psychiat. **113:** 491–494.
29. GITTLESON, N. L. & S. LEVINE. 1966. Subjective ideas of sexual change in male schizophrenics. Brit. J. Psychiat. **112:** 779–782.
30. HABER, R. N., Ed. 1968. Contemporary Theory and Research in Visual Perception. Holt, Rinehart & Winston. New York.
31. HAMILTON, V. 1963. Size constancy and cue responsiveness in psychosis. Brit. J. Psychol. **54:** 25–39.
32. HARRIS, J. G. 1957. Size estimation of pictures as a function of thematic content for schizophrenic and normal subjects. J. Personal. **25:** 651–671.
33. HARWAY, N. I. & L. F. SALZMAN. 1964. Size constancy in psychopathology. J. Abnorm. Soc. Psychol. **69:** 606-613.
34. HELFAND, I. 1956. Role taking in schizophrenia. J. Consult. Psychol. **20:** 37–41.
35. HUSNI-PALACIOS, M., J. R. PALACIOS & P. J. GIBEAU. 1967. Auditory perceptual patterns of process and reactive schizophrenics. J. Project. Tech. Personal. Assess. **31:** 86–91.
36. ISCOE, I. & D. J. VELDMAN. 1963. Perception of an emotional continuum by schizophrenics, normal adults and children. J. Clin. Psychol. **19:** 272–276.
37. JACKSON, W. & A. C. CARR. 1955. Empathic ability in normals and schizophrenics. J. Abnorm. Soc. Psychol. **51:** 79–82.
38. JOHANSSEN, W. J., S. H. FRIEDMAN & J. V. LICCIONE. 1964. Visual perception as a function of chronicity in schizophrenia. Brit. J. Psychiat. **110:** 561–570.
39. JOHANNSEN, W. J. & R. F. TESTIN. 1966. Assimilation of information: A function of Chronicity in Schizophrenia. Arch. Gen. Psychiat. **15:** 492–498.
40. KELM, H. 1962. The figural after-effect in schizophrenic patients. J. Nerv. Ment. Dis. **135:** 338–345.
41. KELM, H. 1968. Visual figural after-effect in schizophrenic and nonschizophrenic patients. J. Abnorm. Psychol. **73:** 273–275.
42. KIDD, A. H. 1964. Monocular distance perception in schizophrenics. J. Abnorm. Soc. Psychol. **68:** 100–103.

43. KLEIN, G. S. 1951. The personal world through perception. *In* Perception: An Approach to Personality. R. R. Blake & C. V. Ramsey, Eds. : 328–355. Ronald. New York.
44. KOLB, L. C. 1959. Disturbances of the body-image. *In* American Handbook of Psychiatry. S. Arieti, Ed. : 749–769. Basic Books. New York.
45. LANG, P. J. & A. H. BUSS. 1965. Psychological deficit in schizopherenia: II. Interference and activation. J. Abnorm. Psychol. **70:** 77–106.
46. LEVINSON, A. 1966. Auditory hallucinations in a case of hysteria. Brit. J. Psychiat. **112:** 19–26.
47. LOVINGER, E. 1956. Perceptual contact with reality in schizophrenics. J. Abnorm. Soc. Psychol. **52:** 87–91.
48. MCGHIE, A. 1966. Psychological studies of schizophrenia. *In* Studies on Psychosis. T. Freeman, J. L. Cameron & A. McGhie, Eds. : 176–196. International Universities Press. New York.
49. MCGHIE, A. 1966. Psychological studies of schizophrenia. Brit. J. Med. Psychol. **39:** 281–288.
50. MCGINNIES, E. 1949. Emotionality and perceptual defense. Psychol. Rev. **56:** 244–251.
51. MEDNICK, S. A. & T. F. MCNEIL. 1968. Current methodology in research on the etiology of schizophrenia: Serious difficulties which suggest the use of the high-risk-group method. Psychol. Bull. **70:** 681–693.
52. MILGRAM, N. A. 1960. Cognitive and empathic factors in role-taking by schizophrenic and brain-damaged patients. J. Abnorm. Soc. Psychol. **60:** 219–224.
53. MILGRAM, N. A. 1961. Role-taking in female schizophrenic patients. J. Clin. Psychol. **17:** 409–411.
54. MOON, A. F., R. B. MEFFERD, B. A. WIELAND, A. POKORNY & G. A. FALCONER. 1968. Perceptual dysfunction as a determinant of schizophrenic word associations. J. Nerv. Ment. Dis. **146:** 80–84.
55. PAYNE, P. W. 1966. The measurement and significance of overinclusive thinking and retardation in schizophrenic patients. *In* Psychopathology of Schizophrenia. P. H. Hoch & J. Zubin, Eds. : 77–97. Grune & Stratton. New York.
56. PISHKIN, V., T. E. SMITH & H. W. LEIBOWITZ. 1962. The influence of symbolic stimulus value on perceived size in chronic schizophrenia. J. Consult. Psychol. **26:** 323–339.
57. RAUSH, H. L. 1952. Perceptual constancy in schizophrenia. J. Personal. **21:** 176–187.
58. RAUSH, H. L. 1956. Object constancy in schizophrenia: The enhancement of symbolic objects and conceptual stability. J. Abnorm. Soc. Psychol. **52:** 231–234.
59. ROMANO, J., Ed. 1967. The Origins of Schizophrenia. Excerpta Medica Foundation. Amsterdam.
60. ROSENTHAL, D., W. G. LAWLER, T. P. ZAHN & D. SHAKOW. 1960. The relationship of some aspects of mental set to degree of schizophrenic disorganization. J. Personal. **28:** 26–38.
61. SANDERS, R. S. & A. R. PACHT. 1952. Perceptual size constancy of known clinical groups. J. Consult. Psychol. **16:** 440–444.
62. SAUCER, R. T. 1958. A further study of apparent motion of schizophrenics. J. Consult. Psychol. **22:** 256.
63. SEDMAN, G. 1967. Experimental and phenomenological approaches to the problem of hallucinations in organic psycho-syndromes. British J. Psychiat. **113:** 1115–1121.
64. SHAKOW, D. 1962. Segmental set: a theory of the formal psychological deficit in schizophrenia. Arch. Gen. Psychiat. **6:** 1–17.
65. SHAKOW, D. 1963. Psychological deficit in schizophrenia. Behav. Sci. **8:** 275–305.
66. SHAKOW, D. 1967. Understanding normal psychological function: Contributions from schizophrenia. Arch. Gen. Psychiat. **17:** 306–319.
67. SHAKOW, D. 1969. On doing research in schizophrenia. Arch. Gen. Psychiat. **20:** 618–642.
68. SILVERMAN, J. 1964. The problem of attention in research and theory in schizophrenia. Psychol. Rev. **71:** 352–379.
69. SILVERMAN, J. 1964. Scanning-control mechanism and "cognitive" filtering in paranoid and nonparanoid schizophrenia. J. Consult. Psychol. **28:** 385–393.
70. SILVERMAN, J. 1964. Perceptual control of stimulus intensity in paranoid and nonparanoid schizophrenia. J. Nerv. Ment. Dis. **139:** 545–549.
71. SILVERMAN, J. 1967. Variations in the cognitive control and psycho-physiological defense in the schizophrenias. Psychosomat. Med. **29:** 225–251.
72. SNYDER, S. 1961. Perceptual closure in acute paranoid schizophrenics. Arch. Gen. Psychiat. **5:** 406–410.
73. SNYDER, S., D. ROSENTHAL & I. R. TAYLOR. 1961. Perceptual closure in schizophrenia. J. Abnorm. Soc. Psychol. **63:** 131–136.

74. TUCKER, G., M. HARROW, T. DETRE & B. HOFFMAN. 1969. Perceptual experiences in schizophrenic and nonschizophrenic patients. Arch. Gen. Psychiat. **20:** 159–166.
75. TURBINER, M. 1961. Choice discrimination in schizophrenic and normal subjects for positive, negative, and neutral affective stimuli. J. Consult. Psychol. **25:** 92.
76. VENABLES, P. H. 1964. Input dysfunction in schizophrenia. *In* Progress in Experimental Personality Research. Vol. I. B. A. Maher, Ed. : 1–47. Academic Press. New York.
77. VON FIEANDT, K. & M. WERTHEIMER. 1969. Perception. Annual Rev. Psychol. **20:** 159–192.
78. WECKOWICZ, T. E. 1957. Size constancy in schizophrenic patients. J. Ment. Sci. **103:** 475–486.
79. WECKOWICZ, T. E. 1964. Shape constancy in schizophrenic patients. J. Abnorm. Soc. Psychol. **68:** 177–183.
80. WECKOWICZ, T. E. & D. B. BLEWETT. 1959. Size constancy and abstract thinking in schizophrenia. J. Ment. Sci. **105:** 909–934.
81. WECKOWICZ, T. E. & R. HALL. 1960. Distance constancy in schizophrenic and non-schizophrenic mental patients. J. Clin. Psychol. **16:** 272–276.
82. WECKOWICZ, T. E. & R. SOMMER. 1960. Body image and self-concept in schizophrenia. J. Ment. Sci. **106:** 17–39.
83. WECKOWICZ, T. E., R. SOMMER & R. HALL. 1958. Distance constancy in schizophrenic patients. J. Ment. Sci. **104:** 1174–1182.
84. WEINER, H. 1958. Diagnosis and symptomatology. *In* Schizophrenia: A Review of the Syndrome. L. Bellak, Ed. : 107–173. Logos. New York.
85. WEINER, I. B. 1966. Psychodiagnosis in Schizophrenia. Wiley. New York.
86. WERTHEIMER, M. 1954. The differential satiability of schizophrenic and normal subjects: A test of a deduction from the theory of figural after-effects. J. Gen. Psychol. **51:** 291–299.
87. WERTHEIMER, M. & C. W. JACKSON, JR. 1957. Figural aftereffects, "brain modifiability," and schizophrenia: A further study. J. Gen. Psychol. **57:** 45–54.
88. WITKIN, H. A. 1965. Psychological differentiation and forms of pathology. J. Abnorm. Psychol. **70:** 317–336.
89. WITKIN, H. A., R. B. DYK, H. F. FATERSON, D. R. GOODENOUGH & S. A. KARP. 1962. Psychological Differentiation. Wiley. New York.
90. ZAHN, T. P. 1959. Acquired and symbolic affective value as determinants of size estimation in schizophrenic and normal subjects. J. Abnorm. Soc. Psychol. **58:** 39–47.

DISCUSSION

DR. CRAWFORD CLARK (*New York State Psychiatric Institute and Columbia University*): I'd like to question to what extent, in all of your data and all of the studies you reported, these differences represent only a difference in response bias between the patient and control, rather than a difference in sensory sensitivity or perception. This goes back to Diamond in 1958, who pointed out in the perceptual defense studies, that the social penalty for reporting a taboo word at present, when the experimenter had presented an innocent word, is very high. Therefore, subjects are very cautious; they want to be very certain, before pronouncing it, that a taboo word was indeed present before they say that they heard it.

At that time Diamond wasn't aware of, or only slightly aware of, a signal detection theory which permits a distinction to be made between sensory sensitivity deprime and response bias, that is, the criterion that the subject uses, or, as they call it, the likelihood ratio.

In our own work we have found differences in threshholds, using the method of limits, between hospitalized patients and normal controls. However, when we subject these reports to a signal detection theory analysis, we find no differences between patients and normals with respect to sensory sensitivity. There is, however, a difference in response bias. Patients are very cautious about reporting the presence of something. And this makes sense in a hospital setting: the patient reports that something is not there, that is, he gives a yes response to a blank—he's reporting hallucinations. As with the taboo word, there is a high social penalty here. These social penalties are influencing response bias, and there is actually no difference in the sensory sensitivity.

We've not been able to find any differences so far in between patients and normals. All the differences are response bias. A contrasting study a little bit more optimistic is that by Price and Erickson. They used size constancy, I believe, comparing schizophrenics, paranoid schizophrenics, and, I think, normal controls.

Using traditional procedures to analyze the data, they found no difference in size constancy. However, when they did use a signal detection theory approach to analyze the data, they did find some differences.

DR. WEINER: These are very important points which have by no means been resolved. In the study planned at this point in time I took into account such development as far as research strategy, in trying to evaluate older literature. It's always a question in terms of what is going to be construed as raw data. The subject is giving some response that can be assessed at a phenomenological level. You decide what it is you're going to measure. It may be a movement, an action, or a self-report, or a "yes" or "no" report, and you may be sure, particularly looking back and reviewing other studies, how accurately that reflected what the person actually was thinking or sensing at that time. There may be many reasons why the phenomenological data would differ from what we might call the actual data, depending on our philosophy, which I don't want to get into right now. I only wish to point out that this is particularly significant with regard to studies of schizophrenia. And I can speak more knowledgeably about research on schizophrenia than I can on perception. But there is a host of variables that seem clearly to influence how schizophrenics will respond in an experimental setting, independently of their particular talents or abilities in connection with what is being measured.

The aspect of being a patient and concern about report would be another variable. But for schizophrenics it's a whole context of an interpersonal examination situation, as proved to be significant in many studies. Many schizophrenic patients have particular concerns about their relationships with people. They have more difficulty relative to various control groups than in interacting with an examiner with regard to some cognitive task, so that differences can be demonstrated in schizophrenic performance on cognitive measures.

There are differences between a task that's administered by examiners who are physically present, and a task that's administered by a machine that flashes buttons and responses in terms of some quoted response with no other physical presence. These are important issues, any many of them are difficult to resolve, going back and looking at studies that have been done both in design and because you can't really tell what the actual experience was, especially if your approach is to define actual experience as being something other than the observed behavior, or the phenomena that would be observably judged or by anyone participating in the research.

UNIDENTIFIED SPEAKER: I would like to ask the following question. All the data that you reported relative to schizophrenics. How do neurotics, for example, react in situations in which they are asked to estimate size, body parts? Are they similar to the normals? Or are they more like neurotics or psychotics?

DR. WEINER: I think there are a number of answers to that, depending on the kind of literature one looks at generally in terms of this kind. The study of the neurotic has been a rather overlooked group, perhaps for a number of reasons, but the bulk of research is certainly on, if not schizophrenics, some other psychotic group, or organic group compared to some control samples. The latter may be normal samples, or may be another clinical sample that is nonschizophrenic, so neurotics are perhaps included and aren't identified as such. However, in some studies I mentioned, neurotics had been looked at, particularly with regard to the body experience, for example, Fisher discovered that many neurotic subjects report similar kinds of distorted body perceptions, as the schizophrenics do.

In some studies that have been done in our department on constancy and other perceptual studies, particularly looking at subgroups of neurotic patients as clearly as they can be defined in terms of how effective our diagnostic discriminations are, neurotically depressed patients, or patients with anxiety or hysterical types of neuroses seem to differ from normal subjects and also from schizophrenic subjects, and it seems to be quite variable.

UNIDENTIFIED SPEAKER: From your answer to Dr. Clark, I got the queasy feeling that we're in no better a state today than we ever have been, in terms of defining our terms and establishing comparable standards of measurement, so that one experiment can be compared to another. Am I correct in this, or are we moving towards some kind of mutual understanding in the field in trying to understand the concepts and the phenomena that we're trying to measure, even if we don't know what schizophrenia is, or what a perception is, or what a sensation is? Do we not yet have a method by which to establish conventional standards for describing phenomena and then try to measure them the same way so that we can come out with some data that are comparable and understandable from one decade to another and from one clinical field to another? As a clinician, I will find it very hard to use the material so far educed today.

DR. WEINER: I can respond to that in two ways. In terms of the experimental design, one that started in terms of what is schizophrenia, how do we identify subject groups for research purposes? Now there is a question regarding the tremendous literature on the unreliability of diagnostic groups and problems of nosology. Some investigators insist that they can't make any reasonable diagnoses and, hence, we can't study these phenomena. But there are others who take a much different point of view, strongly asserting that developing adequate nosology and ways of identifying subject groups is an essential prerequisite to doing meaningful research on psychopathology. Dr. Lorr has presented one major research approach to this in terms of establishing certain syndromes that have some relationship, although not equivalent to more traditional nomenclature, but based on some kind of system of measurement that can be used consistently to identify the same group for research purposes.

Now, let me leave the diagnostic problem aside. Now at the other end, the problem is in regard to the whole approach to research in terms of construct validity, which is, at times, a bit vague in concept. However we do have some clinical notions of what schizophrenia is, and what kinds of disturbances, or cognitive deficits, or whatever, characterize it. And if there are research studies in different places and different ways that seem to converge in certain ways, then we start to get the feeling that we do know something about what these phenomena are, and if they are consistent with the theoretical ideas of what schizophrenia is, we assume that the people we sampled and studies have some kinds of schizophrenic disturbance. I think that one of the strongest convergences of such a research approach is one that I refer to today concerning an interference approach to schizophrenia. The concept that the essential disturbance in schizophrenia is a basic inability to pay attention, or to maintain a relevant focus of attention. This convergence has come from many different points of view, many different laboratories, a wide range of experimental designs, and also from people who have much different views on what the etiology this disturbed attentional state might be, in terms of a deficit or neurological organization or a deficit in early interpersonal relationship, or whatever. I feel that it has given us to date probably the most powerful underfstanding of the phenomenas of schizophrenia, that is, this kind of interference or attentional deficit notion.

MARCIA RABINOWITZ (*N.Y.U. Medical Center, N. Y.*): In the reports that you mentioned, I'd like to ask whether these research studies took place on adults only, or whether children were included, or whether there is some special research about children? I'm sure there is. And if so, have children who have been diagnosed as schizophrenic been found to be different clinical entities from adults?

DR. WEINER: I think that perhaps all, or almost all, of the studies that I referred to, or reviewed without mentioning but which aren't included, are based on adult subjects, primarily. So far, I think studies of children as such haven't contributed that much generally to the literature on cognitive deficit in schizophrenia. They've contributed more to ideas about child development and, also in the whole area of developmental psychopathology, for the last couple of years, there's been a major shift, among people interested in psychopathology, from comparing adult groups toward studying children, particularly on longitudinal studies, so that I think the main contribution from that area is yet to come.

I think that there are a number of observations on childhood schizophrenia from the clinical point of view, and most of these would suggest that when the childhood schizophrenic becomes an adult, he is primarily similar to the chronic long-term adult schizophrenic.

Part IV. Perception of Creativity

THE PERCEPTION OF OBJECTS OF ART

Carroll C. Pratt

Princeton University, Princeton and Rider College, Trenton, N. J.

Peripheral sensory stimulation that leads to the perception of the external world is little more than a meaningless pattern of hieroglyphics. When the hieroglyphics are then transmitted to the sensorium by electrochemical explosions along the nerve fibers, they surely bear no resemblance whatever to three-dimensional objects of all kinds of shapes and sizes and various distances in space. The head, eyes and ears are, moreover, in frequent movement; yet the perceived world retains a remarkable stability and constancy. The objects in a room seem to stay put no matter in what direction or how rapidly the eyes move. A man 20 feet away appears to be about the same size as a man standing nearby, although the retinal images of the person looking at the men are quite different in size.

When confronted with manifold mysteries such as these, Helmholtz came to the conclusion that the apparent stability of the perceived world is the result of past experience. From infancy on, the blooming, buzzing sensory confusions acquire more or less fixed meanings which then serve to keep objects in their proper place. Experience translates the hieroglyphics into recognizable chairs, tables, books, windows, staircases, and people. Men at different distances are still recognized as men and, therefore, judged to be about the same size. Most of our waking hours we are in the presence of familiar sights and sounds, and their mnemonic traces or engrams have long since acquired a life tenure. When the engrams are subexcited by what was originally a meaningless pattern of hieroglyphics, the attendant response is swift and sure and, usually, surprisingly accurate. We sit down on chairs, close doors, make knots in our ties and shoestrings, carry on conversations, punch keys on a typewriter, run up and down stairs, and even steer an automobile through heavy traffic with hardly a scratch. The mind makes an *unbewusster Schluss*, to use Helmholtz's phrase, an unconscious inference that makes it possible for past experience to present us with a perceived world in which we ordinarily find our way about with no trouble at all. It rarely occurs to us that things are not what they seem, or that what we see and hear cannot possibly correspond with sensory stimulation or external stimuli.

This doctrine of Helmholtz, often referred to as empiricism in perception, has dominated psychological thinking right down to the present day. In this country this view was most clearly and forcefully expounded by the late Edward Bradford Titchener of Cornell University. For Titchener perceptions always have meaning, and in his system meaning is a context built up by past experience that accrues to the core of sensations. Sensations do not mean anything. They are sensory elements that are described in terms of their attributes of quality, duration, intensity, and extensity. When a context is added on to the sensations, then the core has a meaning: It is a book, a house, an automobile, and so forth; and it is always something more than is delivered to the sensorium by sensory stimulation. Perception is a meaning, not just an aggregate of sensations.

Titchener's rather extreme and dogmatic empiricism is well illustrated in his treatment of the perception of distance. The hieroglyphics on the retina are formed on a bidimensional surface, and it was taken for granted by Titchener that they therefore could not possibly furnish a clue to three dimensions. The fact that we nevertheless see objects in tridimensional space is consequently an antinomy that psychology must somehow try to solve. There is no sensory clue to three dimensions, yet perceived distance is as palpable as anything can be. Why? "We seem," said Titchener, "quite immediately and directly to see distances; we see that our friend is coming nearer, we see that he has passed the bridge, we see when to shake hands with him. Yet there is no sensation of distance, and there is no specific stimulus to distance. What then really happens?"

What happens, Titchener goes on to say, is that a context of kinesthetic and visual sensations and images accrues to the bidimensional core and confers on it the *meaning* of distance. Distance is a learned illusion, as it were, which, since early life, has become a *brain habit*–to use Titchener's favorite phrase for past experience. Titchener concedes that learning is a psychological problem, but that the actual things learned are matters to be dropped into the epistemological wastebasket.

The quotation from Titchener is taken from a book first published in 1915, and remains unaltered in subsequent editions.[1] He had expressed similar views many times before in other publications, so it may be assumed that he remained faithful throughout his life to the doctrine of perception which he first learned under Wundt during his student days in Leipzig. His only addition was the elaboration of his well-known context theory of meaning which placed practically all psychological events above the level of sensation in the casket of past experience.

By 1915 behaviorism and Gestalt psychology had already appeared on the scene, but their influence was not felt until after the war. Perception, as treated by classical psychology, was ignored by behaviorism because it had the taint of subjectivism which was anathema to the early radicals. For Gestalt psychology, however, perception occupied the very center of the stage and remained there throughout the lives of the triumvirate–Wertheimer, Koffka, and Köhler. These men swung the pendulum back to nativism which had been rather ambiguously espoused by Hering, a contemporary of Helmholtz, but which failed to gain more than a small handful of adherents during the next half century or more. It may be said as a rough generalization that nativism, in contrast to empiricism, assumes that perception depends on external stimuli, sensory stimulation, and the characteristics of brain structure, and that past experience plays an insignificant role.

Innumerable studies done by the Gestalt psychologists and published in their journal, *Psychologische Forschungen,* were designed to show that the perceived world depends less on past experience than on sensory stimulation and field forces in the brain. Gottschaldt's well-known experiment is a good example.[2] Observers were made familiar with various geometrical designs by so many presentations that each one could be identified without any hesitation or error. The designs were then presented in the context of a larger shape made by the addition of lines of one kind or another, but the original design was still there exactly as it had first been learned. The observers were told to find the original design. Gottschaldt argued that familiarity by repeated exposures, i.e., past experience, should make the original designs spring forth, as it were, for easy recognition. Such was not the case. Most of the observers had great difficulty in finding the designs, and some of them could not locate the designs at all, in spite of the many times they had been exposed to them. Past experience was of no avail. *Quod erat demonstrandum.*

The foremost student of perception in this country today is undoubtedly James

J. Gibson of Cornell University. After his graduate studies at Princeton, Gibson came under the influence of Koffka, and from that time on his views have been much closer to Gestalt psychology than to the doctrines he learned in his earlier student days. He has parted company with the Gestalt psychologists in some respects, especially in their physiological speculations which he considers of dubious value; but he resembles them in his insistence that perception is neither a bundle of sensations nor a product of past experience, except in certain very special cases. His experimental studies have been referred to as a global psychophysics, a search for stimulus-correlates of the total perceptual object, the *Gestalten*, if you will, just as Fechner's work made possible a quantitative statement of the relation between stimulus and sensation. If stimulus-correlates of perception can be found—and Gibson has discovered many new and important ones—then it is unnecessary to make any appeal to past experience to account for perception. One example of what Gibson has done in this regard must suffice.[3]

We have already seen that Titchener looked upon the perception of distance as a meaning, a type of learned illusion. Now let us look at the way Gibson deals with the same problem. Distance is not a simple sensory attribute, nor is it an acquired meaning; and least of all is it an illusion, unless one wants to argue that the whole phenomenal world is an illusion, in which case the problem for psychology still remains: How does it happen that the only world we know anything about appears the way it does? How does stimulation on a bidimensional retina produce impressions of objects in three-dimensional space?

FIGURE 1 shows one aspect of Gibson's global psychophysics.[3] Objects A, B, C, and D are at different distances in a line extending straight outward from the eye. If these objects happen to be dimly illuminated discs seen through a reduction screen in a pitch dark tunnel, both their distance and size are indeterminate. They may be seen as small discs near at hand or as large discs far away. But viewing objects in this way is artificial and unreal. In everyday perception all objects at various distances in front of an observer are seen over a longitudinal surface, and on that surface or ground, are points or highlights created by innumerable kinds of texture, edges, lines, changes in brightness, ripples and waves, boards, bricks, parked automobiles, and so forth. Points W, X, Y, and Z are at distances that correspond with A, B, C, and D; and these points on the ground form discriminable gradients on the retina. The gradients are *correlates* of distance. The retinal gradient *wx* is larger than *yz* and thus serves as a clue that A and B are nearer than C and D. Perceived objects need not *resemble* their physical correlates any more than red looks like 650 mμ or middle C sounds like 256 cycles. These

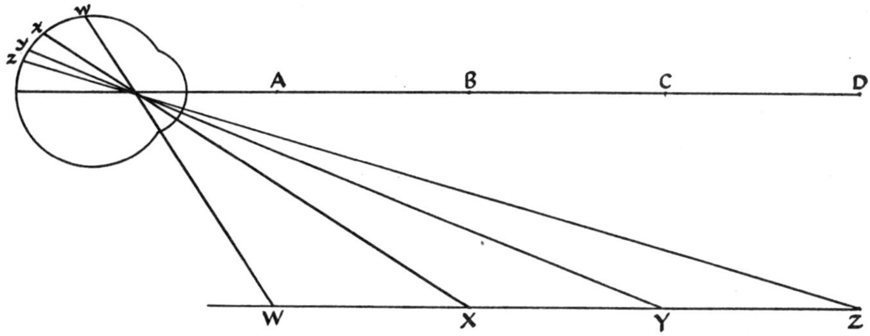

FIGURE 1. Two formulations of the problem of perceived distance. (from Gibson,[3] p. 62.)

stimulus frequencies are *correlates*, not representations of hue and pitch.

The point of view of global psychophysics rests on the assumption that the psychological events under investigation are correlated with stimulus variables. If this correlation can be demonstrated, then an appeal to meaning, past experience, or any other "something more" concept is abandoned in favor of an adherence to a "nothing but" principle of covariation. Gibson has assembled impressive evidence that a "nothing but" principle goes a long way toward accounting for the complexities of perception that an older psychology, beginning with Helmholtz' *unbewusster Schluss*, had only been able to deal with by dragging in all sorts of elusive and often meaningless concepts designed to supplement the small core of perception that is stimulus-bound. The newer nativism in perception seeks to show that a large and important segment that formerly was regarded as meaning, if not illusion, is also stimulus-bound.

The probability that a large part of perception is stimulus-bound has had a profound influence in certain areas of the philosophy and psychology of art. Objects of art are obviously important items in the world of perception, so that any marked change in perceptual theory would presumably have an effect, after some cultural lag, in the field of esthetics, which is exactly what has happened.

The Gestalt psychologists, especially Köhler, frequently refer to qualities of perception rarely dealt with in earlier studies in this area. A face may be remembered and easily recognized as cheerful and friendly, although the shape of the face, the color of the hair and eyes, or the size of the nose and ears are only dimly recalled. A room appears inviting and hospitable, a street dingy and drab, the waves of the sea tempestuous, a landscape soft and tranquil.

These qualities are frequently much more striking in the perception of works of art. Indeed many authorities regard them, by whatever name they may be called, as the very essence of the tenacious hold that art has had in all times and places over the minds of men. The sculpture of Michelangelo and the music of Beethoven often reveal a titanic power, although both have moments of gentle tenderness. The Renaissance madonnas are invariably wistful and even a bit sad. In the right light the glass of Chartres fairly dances with radiance. The color in many of Rembrandt's paintings is somber and at times almost forbidding. Beneath the elegant and often exuberant surface of Mozart's eternally youthful music one may detect a plaintive melancholy, a subdued inner voice that, in combination with the sprightly surface, produces a miracle that many insist is equalled nowhere else in the whole realm of art.

Where do such qualities come from? What is their place in the psychology of perception? In the traditional study of perception they were either ignored or turned over with more or less indifference to Lipps's doctrine of empathy or to Santayana's elaboration of his famous statement that "Beauty is pleasure regarded as the quality of an object." Lipps's doctrine of empathy is better known, at least among psychologists, chiefly because the author first made use of it in his studies of visual illusions and then carried it over into the field of esthetics. He and Santayana have one important point in common. They would agree that to call a painting or a piece of music exuberant, for example, is a kind of pathetic fallacy. Such words apply to human moods and feelings, not to objects of perception. If a listener calls a melody sad, it is because the tones subexcite a bit of subjective visceral sadness within him which he then erroneously ascribes to what he hears.

The doctrines of Lipps and Santayana came as godsends at the time they appeared, for they seemed to solve beautifully an ancient baffling problem in esthetics. How do subjective moods and feelings seem actually to be "out there" in the world of art? How can the tones of a melody be sad? Lipps's reply was that, of course, the tones are not sad. They merely seem to be sad by a process of projection. The moods of art are illusory perceptions–*Scheingefühle*, just as for Titchener the perception of distance is a type of learned illusion.

The Gestalt psychologists were among the first critics of empathy. They argued that the doctrine was not only unnecessary; it was in point of fact actually wrong. Lipps would have said that the gracefulness of a line is the result of smooth flowing movements of the eyes, and that an awkward line follows upon jerky eye movements. Accurate studies of eye movements, however, show that they are much the same no matter what surface they scan. It must be, then, that graceful and awkward lines are intrinsic visual qualities, not kinesthetic projections of eye movements. Köhler has said somewhere that he greatly enjoyed the lovely and graceful ballet movements of Pavlova, but that he himself could not possibly have had even the faintest incipient traces of such bodily motions in himself to project into what he was looking at, as the theory of empathy would demand.

The moods perceived in art, or in any kind of perception, were referred to by the Gestalt psychologists as tertiary qualities.[4] These qualities are regarded as intrinsic *Gestalten* present in every sense department. If their appearance in visual and auditory modalities is derived from kinesthetic or organic projections, the problem is then merely pushed back to the question of how they happen to exist in the bodily senses and not in vision and audition. The difficulty vanishes completely if it can be shown, as the Gestalt psychologists have done, that tertiary qualities are present in all sense departments, even more vividly perhaps in vision and audition than elsewhere.

The ease and accuracy with which tertiary qualities are identified in matching experiments indicate, if they do not unequivocally prove, how closely these qualities are bound to the external objects of art, to the manner in which colors, shapes and sounds are put together by the artist. Numerous reports are in the literature of matching haphazard presentations of works of art with haphazard presentations of adjectives that experts have chosen as the best descriptions of the moods, the tertiary qualities.[5] The matchings are invariably way above chance, which would hardly be the case if the listeners were making the matches on the basis of their past experience or empathic projections, for these would presumably vary considerably from individual to individual. There must be something coercive about the nature of the external objects that leads to such uniform judgments regarding the moods which they present.

The doctrine of empathy argues that these moods have their origin in the person listening to or looking at the works of art. It was not Bach who injected such power and majesty into his fugues, nor Beethoven who found the means of expressing sublime moods in some of his later string quartets. It is you and I who perform those miracles. It is we who are responsible for the romantic *Sturm und Drang* in Brahms's trios. It is for us to blush, not for Wagner to be embarrassed, when the indecent exposures of the *Liebestod* sound forth from the stage and orchestra pit. Tonal design cannot be erotic, nor serene, nor sublime. These qualities have their origin in the viscera of the listener, and are projected by him into the auditory perceptions. The composer is not an artist. He is a trained technician, at times an amazing magician, who cleverly manipulates pitch and rhythm. After he has put his notes together, all he can do is sit back and wait until the artistic geniuses in the audience create out of his tonal design the masterpieces which in his innocence or vanity he probably assumed he himself had contrived. Such are the weird implications of empathy in esthetics and the correlative debasement of the role of the artist. The recent attacks on the doctrine of empathy have made an important contribution to the philosophy of art by revealing the clouded perceptions of writers as far back as Plato who have failed to understand what the artist really does.

The concept of tertiary qualities, powerfully reinforced by Gibson's treatment of perception as stimulus-bound, restores to the artist his rightful place among the gods of mankind. It was *Botticelli* whose brush created the sadness in the faces of his madonnas. It was *Palestrina* whose pen wrote tonal designs of unworldly concord. For nearly four centuries what they did has been here to enjoy by those with eyes to see and ears to hear.

References

1. TITCHENER, E. B. 1915. A Beginner's Psychology. p. 126. The Macmillan Company. New York.
2. GOTTSCHALDT, K. 126. Über den Einfluss der Erfahrung auf die Wahrnehmung von Figuren. Psychologische Forschung. : 1–87.
3. GIBSON, J. J. 1954. The Perception of the Visual World. p. 62. Houghton Mifflin Company. Boston.
4. PRATT, C. C. 1962. Tertiary qualities. Psychologische Beiträge. : 365–372; 1961. Aesthetics. Annual Review of Psychology. : 71–92.
5. PRATT, C. C. 1950. Music as the Language of Emotion. Library of Congress, Washington.

Discussion

ARNOLD HYMENN (*New York City*): How does one account for the consensual validation, that is, so much agreement that you know they do attribute such qualities to the art?

DR. PRATT: The agreement among observers is the remarkable thing because it it were past experience, I should think there would be considerable disagreement, empathic projections and past experience are pretty unreliable, as far as agreement goes. I think the advantage of the gestalt theory and Gibson's really is that their views show that the characteristics are stimulus-bound and not internal projections.

ARTHUR WILNER (*Hillside Hospital*): Have there been any studies in regard to this material that dealt with populations from different cultures? Do Chinese people react in the same way as Europeans to these a-pairing stimuli?

DR. PRATT: Yes, but there ought to be a great many more. There are some that can now be found in journals. This is an extremely important question because the first criticism often raised is that students have been brought up in Western culture and they know what kinds of words are used for painting and music. A student of mine had an idea. He got possession of some records from an expert in New York that demonstrated music from the most exotic places all over the world. And he suggested taping a few measures and presenting these weird sounds to our Western ears to see what we would say, using the adjectives given to us by experts who seemed to know what they meant. I haven't got the results here. I heard the records, which I thought were difficult to interpret, but, nevertheless, we gave them to the students, and much to my amazement, they came way above chance again. If two things were called, one a lament and the other a military call, they scored correctly immediately. There have been other studies, but this should be looked into further, because the basic assumption would be that if a person feels happy in New York, a person who is in the wilds of the Maori ought to feel somewhat the same way when he's happy.

CONCLUDING REMARKS

Margaret E. Tresselt, Ph.D. and Ernest Harms, Ph.D.

The purpose of this conference was to present the various approaches that have been made and are being made to the wide area of perception. A two-day conference is, of course, too limited a period to cover any one approach with any more than a cursory look and too limited to touch all approaches.

The first three papers were grouped under the title "Perception of the Outer World." Doctors Mayzner and Tresselt gave a brief survey of their new discoveries, sequential blanking and displacement, in the field of visual perception. By using a computer-based cathode-ray tube display system, they have been able to present stimuli at input rates varying from 50 μsec per input to 200 msec per input and up to 100 discrete inputs, which has previously been impossible due to equipment limitations. They also suggest a theoretical model to account for many of their findings. Doctor Walker presented his research work relating stimulus complexity, psychological complexity and preference. He used Tartan Plaid patterns; classical, romantic and baroque architecture for his research with human beings, and used compartments of gray, horizontal lines, vertical lines and checkerboards, or varied the number of buffers in a puzzle box for the animal subjects. The multidimensional analysis reveals challenging interaction effects that open new and different aspects of perception. Doctor Helson called for the reexamination of the Gestalt approach and, by analyzing various experiments in the light of the Adaptation Level Theory, was able to stress the importance of the organism when faced with a judgmental situation.

The second session was labeled "Perception of the Inner World." Doctor Henderson opened this portion, choosing to discuss two aspects of inner perception: the psychological function and the contents of our inner perceptions. Both introverted sensation and intuition could be said to comprise the function of the inner world, whereas the contents themselves can be classified as personal unconscious, cultural unconscious, primordial unconscious, and the unconscious beyond imagery. Doctor Boernstein took a slightly different approach by taking issue with the classical schism between "perceiving" as such and "thinking" as such. Both these functions are interrelated and in line with this viewpoint, he proceeded to provide experimental support. Doctor Spiegel elaborated in detail the clinical significance of the relationship between the perceptual self and the cognitive self (among others), and also discussed the relation of self to the ego.

The third session was introduced under the rubric of "Perception in Abnormal Psychological Experience." Doctor Lorr attempted to indicate the role of perception in identifying psychopathology. By taking various syndromes and utilizing amultivariate analysis, he evaluated the major psychotic and neurotic syndromes and further identified those which may or may not be helped by therapy. Doctor Wolstein discussed the changes that have been taking place from the original Freudian concept and Freud's cultural setting to the present time. He made it evident how much perceptual insight could and does help psychoanalytic inquiry. Doctor Weiner selected very practical, rather than theoretical, problems, by discussing the schizophrenic. Without doubt the schizophrenics are more likely to misperceive themselves and their environment than do "control" subjects. He attempted to delineate attentional states and cognitive disposition which would affect their perceptual functioning. "Perception of Creativity" was the last topic to be discussed and was perhaps one of the most challenging. Doctor Mowrer presented a paper* on perception and the learning and uses of language, starting the discussion with a challenge about whether the psychology of perception or phenomenology can make a contribution to the psychology of language. The confusion in the field of psycholinguistics is great, and he seemed to minimize the importance of sense perception. On the other hand, Doctor Pratt offered a survey of the perceptual aspect of esthetics. The contribution of the demonstrations of Ames, the gradients emphasized by Gibson, and the doctrine of empathy suggested by Lipps were considered separately. The relationship of the viewer of a painting or listener to a tune is more than just the organismic qualities or the external stimuli; it is a combination of these which should be investigated still further.

In brief, then, the conference attempted the mammoth task of sampling problems in perception and discussing the role of perception in information processing, in the clinical setting, in the abnormal mind, and in the arts. Each area has its own problems, its own significance, and its own methodology and theory. It was clear that each aspect was incomplete, the entire field requiring a great deal more research.

* Due to circumstances beyond his control, Dr. Mowrer was unable to include his contribution in the monograph.

Printed in the United States of America